THE COURAGE TO TURN INWARD: WHISPERS FROM THE SELF

A Memoir of Healing, Integration, and Becoming Whole

by Hana

Disclaimer

This book reflects my personal experiences, reflections, and perspectives on healing, growth, and self-discovery. It is not intended to provide professional advice, counseling, psychotherapy, or medical treatment. While I am a social worker, this work is written in my capacity as an author.

The content of this book is for informational and inspirational purposes only. It should not be relied upon as a substitute for professional help. Readers are encouraged to seek the support of a qualified mental health professional, medical provider, or other appropriate resource if they are in need of therapeutic care or assistance.

This memoir does not share names, identifying details, and certain circumstances in order to protect the privacy of individuals. While readers may draw associations with real people, any such associations are discouraged to avoid affecting innocent individuals.

The author shall **not** be held liable for any loss, harm, or consequences that may arise from the use, application, or interpretation of the material contained in this book.

Copyright © by Hana Mazare
All rights reserved
ISBN: 978-1-0697100-0-0
No part of this book may be reproduced or transmitted in any form without permission in writing from the author.

Acknowledgements

Thank you to my inner child, all my protective parts, my Self, and the Universe for guiding me through the writing of this memoir! I love you all! Without you, I couldn't have revealed to the world the path we took to break free from the cage of unlovability that was built around us from the moment we entered this world.

Writing this memoir wasn't easy. As I worked on my healing, some parts of me longed to share more details about our past, while others felt hesitant and protective. They just needed time, time to reflect, to discern what truly mattered, and decide what they were ready to release into the world. There are parts of my story that remain private. I share here only what feels safe and necessary, trusting that these glimpses of my journey will resonate without revealing every detail. I am kindly asking my readers to honor both my privacy and my healing journey.

Together, we learned to rise by answering the call to heal. And now, every part of me feels worthy of love, eager, open, and excited for all that life may bring from this moment forward.

A special thank you to my generous friend, who has always been by my side giving me her unconditional love! No words can express the gratitude I have for having her in my life!

Table of Contents

Disclaimer
Acknowledgments
Why I wrote this memoir
Introduction

Part I - My Journey Back to Self   1

Chapter 1. Guided by the Seagulls   1
Chapter 2. My Childhood   5
Chapter 3. The New Me   28

    3.1 Healing My Inner Child   34
    3.2 Healing My "In Control" Protector   50
    3.3 Healing My Highly Functioning Protector   57
    3.4 Healing My Risk Manager Protector   65
    3.5 Healing My Warrior Protector   69
    3.6 Healing My Overgiving Protector   75
    3.7 Healing My Inner Critics   82
       3.7.1 Healing My Obedient Protector   84
       3.7.2 Healing My Negotiator Protector   88
       3.7.3 Healing My Underminer Protector   92
       3.7.4 Healing My Destroyer of Ancestral Trauma Protector   94
    3.8 Meeting My Self   97

Part II - Understanding Self-Absorption Through IFS lens   110

Chapter 4. The Internal Landscape of Self-Absorbed People   110

  4.1 The Inner Child of a Self-Absorbed Person   112
  4.2 The "In Control" Protector   125
  4.3 The Chameleon Protector   131
  4.4 The Manipulative Protector   142
  4.5 The Grandiose Protector   154
  4.6 The Inner Critics   169
    4.6.1 The Conformist Inner Critic Protector   171
    4.6.2 The Comparer Protector   174
    4.6.3 The Dependency Critic Protector   177
    4.6.4 The Doubtful Critic Protector   179
  4.7 The Scarcity - Minded Protector   182
  4.8 The Perfectionistic Protector   191
  4.9 The Revengeful Firefighter   196
  4.10 The Cheater Firefighter   204
  4.11 The Self of a Self-Absorbed Person   208

Conclusions   212
Bibliography   216

Why I wrote this memoir

I have folded myself
into the corners of others' lives -
soft, devoted, unseen.
But now, I unfold.
I light the candle inward.
I come home.
The rest of my life
belongs to the one
I abandoned the most:
Me.

"There is no greater agony than bearing an untold story inside you." (1)

This memoir is my way of breaking the silence that has been imposed on me and for anyone who has felt erased, confused, or ashamed because of someone else's manipulation and control. For much of my life, I believed my voice didn't matter, that speaking the truth was dangerous, shameful, or selfish. But untold stories don't disappear. They whisper in your dreams, tighten your chest, haunt your inner child and silence your soul's calling, and live in your relationships. While healing and writing this memoir, I stopped carrying it quietly.

Writing my memoir was part of my healing journey toward self-love. It offers a glimpse of the struggles faced by my inner child since her voice was silenced and her needs were pushed away by her family. For years, she carried the weight of her unspoken wounds, navigating the confusion, pain, and invisibility that so often follow the abuse from self-absorbed people. Though, my memoir is not a record of blame, a way to seek revenge, or just a story of survival. It is a journey of transformation brought by redesigned actions of protection for my inner child, who learned to use her voice; a story of return to myself, a message that healing is possible, and that truth is not too much. My truth isn't something I can just think about or wait for. It reveals itself through the choices I make, the boundaries I hold, the voice I stop silencing, the life I dare to claim. I choose to live my truth - not perfectly, but honestly.

The very essence of the work we need to do to learn to love ourselves lies in this statement:

"Your task is not to seek for love, but merely to seek and find all the barriers within yourself that you have built against it, and embrace them." (2)

Through long stretches of introspection, I have come to realize that at the root of nearly every wound, every repeated pattern, every silent ache from our life stems from lack of self-love. When I stopped letting others define my value, I learned that self-love is the best antidote to abuse from self-absorbed people.

Self-love has a ripple effect on all areas of our lives, as we reclaim full ownership over our destiny.

New doors started opening for me after I started my healing journey and Internal Family Systems Therapy (IFS) has been one of the biggest. Once I realized that my adult problems stemmed from my childhood, I felt inspired to learn more about this therapeutic modality. Learning more about the system of parts inside us that is protecting our inner child, how they function, and about the healing energy of the Self, made sense to me immediately. I came to understand that my inner child had been buried under multiple layers of pain that had held her back most of her life, affecting her ability to thrive as every child is supposed to. As I made a commitment to give myself the gift of a new life, one with less disappointments and pain, I started the daring tasks of recognizing the pain of my inner child, understanding my protective parts, and helping them align with the values of my Self.

After remembering that my Self has always wanted to be free and live in harmony, I made the decision to stop prioritizing the people who left me behind and disregarded my needs. Looking back at my life journey, I recognized that some of the things that bothered me the most in other people revealed my own invisible unhealed wounds. I believe that every painful experience I've endured was divinely placed on my path, not as punishment, but as preparation. These trials were not random; they were meant for me, so that I could learn to discern between truth and illusion, love and manipulation, light and shadow. Life has been my greatest teacher. With clearer vision and a humbled heart, I can offer others the insight and compassion I've gained along the way. I had to learn that it was my responsibility to give love to myself by removing all these people from my life and shift my focus on things that I wanted to build for myself. Ultimately, in my healing journey, I've acknowledged that I have never been alone. I have gradually become aware that we are connected to everything around: human beings, animals, Gaia, and the Universe.

Another door opened for me when I started to read avidly the work of Dr. Frank Anderson, Harvard-trained psychiatrist, lead IFS trainer and a world-renowned trauma expert. I enjoyed reading especially his memoir, *"To be loved"*, which touched my heart and validated some of my own life experiences. Like me, he had two wounded parents who projected onto him their struggles, shaping a good part of his life. His story helped a protective part of me who struggled with the idea of sharing my life story with people who don't know me, as she was concerned about the potential criticism of my audience, thinking that these people could judge me for supporting others at times when I couldn't help myself very well. It gave this part of me permission to remove these concerns after acknowledging that we always evolve. The person I was ten years ago is different from the one I was three years ago, the one I am today and the one I will be five years from now.

Each one has had a unique view upon life and each has helped others in a potentially different way. But no way of helping has been wrong, because each one has tried to help other people out of love .

A few months later, another door opened when I came across the work of Lissa Rankin. I started reading her memoir, *"The Anatomy of a Calling"*. Her memoir validated my recent spiritual experiences and helped a protective part of me that was skeptical. This protective part had moments when she whispered her concern that I, the collective of my internal parts, was losing my mind. But no, after reading Lissa's memoir, I learned that I had similar experiences to other people. I was going through my spiritual awakening.

I truly believe now that nothing happens by chance, as shortly after starting to read her book, I learned about the *"Write to heal"* workshop offered by Lissa Rankin and Dr. Frank Anderson. This workshop teaches people about the healing power of writing, using the creativity of our inner child and protective parts.

If you haven't had any introduction to Internal Family Systems Therapy (IFS), you may need to know that this therapeutic modality is based on the idea that the mind is made up of different categories of parts, or "sub-personalities" exiles, managers and firefighters. Each has valuable qualities and each plays a valuable role within the system. In addition to these parts, there is also the Self, which is the essence within everyone. *Self* is characterized by clarity, compassion, courage, confidence, curiosity, and many other values that vary from person to person. *Exiles* are the aspects of our psyche that hold the joys of our childhood, as well as our sorrows and traumas. Some might be frozen in the past by oppressive practices, hold overwhelming terror, loneliness, sadness, and emptiness that affected their development. The inner child holds beliefs that shape our present perceptions. When exiles are triggered, people become overwhelmed by emotions. *Managers* are the parts of us that aim to keep the system functional and safe. Some of them are potentially present from the beginning of the inner child's life, holding characteristics of people's personality or inherited from our ancestors. They keep unpleasant emotions out of consciousness and, consequently, try to keep the exiles well hidden. If someone has been humiliated, ashamed, or frightened, the managers want to make sure that the exiles won't get too close or dependent on others, who may harm them again. They may also focus on taking care of others rather than looking after their own needs. When the managers fail in their duty to prevent the activation of the exiles, firefighters rush in to do anything they can to put out the flames of the overwhelming emotions. They may engage in self-harming behaviour, binge eating, drug and/or alcohol consumption, and even suicide.

Love is a powerful force that can heal wounds when it's incorporated in one's life. It brings a sense of wholeness, and it arises not from looking outside of ourselves to find happiness or completion, but from bringing calmness within ourselves. The calmness of our mind gives us the confidence to navigate relationships with other people without getting entangled in their negative emotions. When there is conflict in our mind, our body starts signaling that something triggers a response of one of our protective parts or inner child. Our heart might start racing, we might lose our sleep, or we might feel tension in our muscles. If we shine a light on the thoughts that spark our inner storm, we could understand the reason for this fire and find the right solutions that bring calmness again. This awareness comes from connecting with protective parts that emerged during difficult times of our inner child and require attention, validation, kindness, and guidance to navigate a new experience. It gives us the power to respond with intention and avoid getting hurt again.

By bringing these hidden parts of ourselves into awareness, we notice how they interact with each other and the specific steps they take to protect their inner child. All our parts have good intentions, as they all want to protect their inner child, even if some of their strategies are destructive. The awareness of their role and strategies moves them toward the leadership of the Self, who guides them to a more genuine and harmonious inner life, rather than one taken over by different parts.

Breaking free from abuse from self-absorbed people comes with awareness. The second part of my memoir explores archetypes in the context of self-absorbed people through an IFS lens, as I believe that recognizing the specific behaviours displayed by a self-absorbed person and the causes of these kinds of behaviours is an important step towards breaking free. It is my desire to give them hope and encouragement to dream for a better life, not only for themselves, but for their future generations. Chaos and collapse could be catalysts for awakening if we choose not to replay old cycles.

Rather than writing this memoir from a single, unified voice, I chose to give voice to my inner child and Self. My inner child speaks with vulnerability and honesty about her pain and longing, while my Self - the calm, compassionate core of who I am - shares about her protective parts' roles, perspectives, and their strategies to keep her safe, along with the burdens they've carried for so long. My Self also offers insight, support, and wisdom in their healing journey. Together, they reflect not just a story of survival, but a journey toward wholeness. Through their distinct voices, they explore their roles, thoughts, emotions, and the hopes they now carry for the future.

Everything I've written in this memoir is rooted in lived experience. As a survivor of abuse caused by self-absorbed people, I know firsthand the confusion, isolation, emotional toll it takes, the deep wounds it leaves on the spirit, and the profound strength it takes to reclaim one's light. In my professional calling, I've held space for many who have endured the same struggles, witnessing their courage as they rise from the shadows of self-absorbed people. This memoir is a testimony that pain can be transformed and a reminder that healing is not only possible but divinely guided.

May these pages offer you the same thing I had to fight for: clarity, courage, and the deep knowing that your story, too, deserves to be told.

Introduction

The waves of love that wash over our hearts when we bring a child into this world are unlike anything else - they awaken a strength within us that empowers us to face whatever challenges arise as we nurture and prepare this new life for its journey. Life is not meant to be easy, but it isn't meant to be unbearably difficult either. Much of the hardship we face is created by us - by the collective human experience shaped over generations. When we are burdened by the unconscious wounds and limiting beliefs of those who came before us, we begin to see life through their distorted lens. We unknowingly continue their legacy, passing on their fears and patterns to the children we love so deeply. Ancestral imprints of abandonment, scarcity, and the fear of not belonging often ripple through our lives, closing our hearts to love - love for ourselves, for our children, for those who are different from us, for the Earth, and for the beauty that surrounds us. But healing begins with awareness. And when we choose to open our hearts again, we begin to break the cycle.

The existence of ancestral trauma may be unknown to many of us, yet there is not a single person untouched by its influence. Our ancestors endured unimaginable hardships - wars, famine, oppression, displacement - and often had no choice but to suppress their pain to survive. In doing so, many became disconnected from their true Selves, burying wounds so deep that they echoed silently through generations. These unhealed traumas didn't disappear; they were passed down, subtly shaping how we see ourselves, how we love, how we trust, and how we respond to life. Acknowledging this inheritance is the first step toward breaking the cycle and remembering who we truly are beneath it all.

Ancestral trauma lives in us, in our body, mind, and spirit. It is directly and indirectly shaping our reality, influencing all our interactions if we don't acknowledge its existence and try to heal the wounds that have been handed to us. Healing the wounds of our ancestors requires a strong desire to differentiate from them by reviewing the library of thoughts from our mind and choosing to act from that moment on, only based on the values and beliefs that represent us. Ancestral work involves releasing the pain of our ancestors from our body by developing a better relationship with the container of our emotions. Huge progress in our healing can be made when we connect with our Selves, who are wisely guiding us, showing us every step of the path we need to take to free ourselves from pain.

I wrote this memoir for myself first of all, for my son, who I love very much, and other people who suffered parental abandonment that resulted in cycles of unhealthy relationships during their adulthood. Some of them are survivors of abuse from self-absorbed people, who have faced the devastating effects of many types of abuse, including verbal, emotional, physical, sexual, financial, psychological and spiritual. They have lived life-threatening situations, betrayal, confusion, and isolation that have damaged their sense of safety and identity. The survivors of abuse from self-absorbed people struggle with cognitive dissonance, intrusive thoughts, difficulty trusting themselves, and learned helplessness. It is very difficult to break free from this mental fog, but it's not impossible.

This book is inspired by the Internal Family Systems model, but is not written from a position of IFS certification.

Part I – My Journey Back to Self

Chapter 1

Guided by the Seagulls

Sitting on the beach, watching the vast ocean stretch beyond the horizon and the seagulls dance with the wind, I longed for answers; answers that could set me free. Free from the confusion, the pain, and the limiting beliefs that had shaped my sense of self for far too long. I lifted my gaze to the sky, silently pleading for guidance. I asked the seagulls to show me the way, to bring me the mental clarity and strength I so desperately needed. I was standing at a crossroads, where every possible path stirred uncertainty, and the weight of my decisions felt overwhelming.

Inside me, moments of peace were fleeting. Emotional storms, stirred by the relentless voices of doubt, clouded my mind and made it hard to reclaim the power I had once surrendered. And yet, nature held me gently in that moment. The breeze wrapped around me like freedom, whispering that I was not alone. The warm sand welcomed me, as if the Earth itself was inviting me to rest, to surrender into its embrace. The Ocean sang its eternal song, a melody of resilience, reminding me that life, like the tide, always moves forward. The sunlight kissed my face, a quiet promise that love was still possible.

Love does not ask who you have been,
nor weigh the sum of your past mistakes.
It does not tally wounds or keep records of debts,
it simply opens,
again and again,
like the sky surrendering to dawn.

It waits for no perfection,
it does not demand that you shine.
It sees the trembling beneath your voice,
the shadows behind your eyes,
and still, it whispers
You are enough.

Unconditional love is the fire that warms
without burning,
the river that carries
without asking where you've been.
It is the hand that reaches
even when you turn away,
the patience that lingers
when the night stretches long.

It does not bind;
it frees.
It does not cling;
it breathes.
It is not a cage of promises,
but a vast horizon,

where your spirit can unfold
and find its true name.

This love is the seed that grows
even in broken soil,
the song that plays
when silence weighs heavy.
It is the mother who stays
when storms have scattered the world,
the friend who hears the words
you never dared to speak.

It bends with your sorrow,
it rises with your joy.
It sits quietly in the corner
when all you can do is weep,
and when you're ready,
it lifts you gently,
never rushing,
never retreating.

Unconditional love does not say,
"I will love you *if*..."
It says only,
"I love you.
Through the darkness,
through the light,
in your becoming,
in your breaking,
in your silence,
in your song."

It is not earned,
and so it cannot be lost.
It is not bargained,
and so it cannot be stolen.
It simply *is*
the eternal truth
we are all born longing to remember,
the home we return to
when the world forgets our name.

And when you finally see it,
not as something to chase,
but as something already alive within you,
you understand
unconditional love is not only what you receive,
it is what you are,
what you have always been,
what you are here to give.

Chapter 2

My Childhood

She held the world in tender hands,
Found delight in sunlight, in shifting sands.
Her heart reached outward, soft and wide,
For mother, for family, with love that never died.

She laughed at the clouds, danced in the rain,
Saw wonder in simple things, in pleasure and pain.
Her joy was quiet, her smiles discreet,
Yet in every small act, her love was complete.

Though shadows whispered doubt and fear,
Her kind heart sparkled, bright and clear.
Through every harsh word, every unseen slight,
Her laughter and love shone a gentle light.

Even when the world seemed cold and rough,
Her spirit proved that love and joy were enough.

Acknowledging the hidden influence of my ancestors' unhealed wounds, patterns that silently shaped my thoughts, feelings and actions was deeply painful, but that pain marked the beginning of a new life. It became the threshold to a journey of self-discovery. Through deep introspections, I uncovered layers of unresolved trauma that had been buried in my body and mind for decades. By bringing the unconscious into the light, I made space for true healing. This awareness allowed me to reclaim authorship over my life and to finally release the burdens carried by my inner child and her protective parts, burdens she had held in silence for far too long.

This journey led me into experiences far beyond the ordinary. Along the way, I encountered moments of transcendence, awe, and an unexpected sense of connection with something greater than myself, something that felt like the Universe gently guiding me home.

As a social worker, I've supported survivors of abuse and worked in shelters where women fled unsafe relationships, but I've also lived through abuse from self-absorbed people myself, beginning in childhood. My life has become a continuous learning process, revealing not only the roles I unconsciously played in the lives of those I loved most, but also the painful truth that these people chose, again and again, to hurt me. Learning to recognize this truth has been one of my greatest acts of self-love and healing.

But these learnings didn't arrive all at once - they unfolded slowly, over decades. My healing began a few decades ago, when I made the conscious decision to build my own identity, separate from the one shaped by my family. I felt an urgent need to define my own values and beliefs and become someone beyond the patterns I had inherited. I made progress, though not as quickly as I wished. Considering the type of abuse I endured, how early it began, and the limited resources available in my home country, it's clear to me now that I couldn't have moved any faster. Still, I am deeply grateful for the strength I gained from being on my own since the age of fourteen, even though it was incredibly difficult at the time. I stumbled along the way, but the early steps I made while living in my home country were the foundation of the life I've been building ever since.

After moving to Canada, I was exposed to broader understandings of abuse, oppressive practices, and trauma. Slowly, I began to tolerate the discomfort that comes with setting boundaries, doing less, asking for more, and kindly saying a firm "*no.*" Gradually, I started distancing myself from some of the self-absorbed people in my life. But not all of them. Despite making some meaningful realizations a while ago, I couldn't yet see the whole picture, because parts of me weren't ready.

Healing takes time, and some truths wait for us until we're strong enough to receive them. Consequently, I unintentionally drifted away from my healing journey. It wasn't a conscious decision; I simply hadn't yet learned how to consistently look within, to truly understand my inner world and recognize what I needed to feel safe. I believed I had come far enough to continue growing on my own, but I was wrong. Only when I could no longer deny that my life didn't match the one I yearned for, and when the pain of old wounds began to surface, no longer willing to be buried, did I realize it was time to return to the path. This time, though, I understand something I didn't before: healing isn't a destination. It's a lifelong journey, one that continues to evolve as I do.

Healing from the abuse of self-absorbed people can feel like wandering through a cold, dark forest. In this forest, the echoes of past voices surround you - some sharp and piercing, others soft but haunting. Their sounds overlap, creating a fog of ambiguity and confusion. You long to find a way out, escape the darkness and the pain, to reach the light. There's a powerful urge to trace those voices, find their source and make sense of them. But deep down, you know that doing so would only keep you trapped, circling endlessly through the same shadows.

You begin to question everything - your memory, your instincts, even your sense of reality. In this forest, faces are obscured and trust is elusive. And yet, in that deep and heavy darkness, you come to a crossroads. You can either see the forest as a terrifying place that keeps you tethered to the illusions and wounds of your past - or you can choose to make it a place of refuge, a space where healing can begin.

The turning point came when I realized that only in the darkness of the forest could I truly find the light. I chose to own the forest. And in owning it, the light revealed itself. As I stopped running and instead turned inward, intentionally seeking the echoes of those voices and tracing the impact they had on my sense of self, the forest slowly began to transform. The tangled paths cleared. The sun began to rise, little by little.

True healing required me to break down the distorted reflections cast onto me by others - reflections shaped by their own unresolved trauma. Through revisiting my memories, I began peeling away the layers of pain that had quietly settled in my mind and body over the years. Beneath it all, I uncovered the core of who I truly am. As Carl Jung so wisely said, *"Until you make the unconscious conscious, it will direct your life and you will call it fate."*(3) For me, healing has meant bringing light to the unconscious, and reclaiming the path that was always mine to walk.

Over the years, some of my protective parts took it upon themselves to suppress the painful memories of my inner child. They believed that burying the past was the only way to survive, the only way to move forward. But now, something has shifted. This time, all my parts came together with tenderness and intention. They extended a gentle invitation to my inner child, encouraging her to use her voice and share the memories she had carried in silence for so long. She held the truth of my childhood, and when those long-buried memories began to surface, the pain that emerged was overwhelming. It hit my protective parts harder than they had ever expected. As she brought each memory forward, wound after wound rose to the surface - wounds that had silently fractured her sense of safety, trust, and belonging. And yet, in that pain, there was also the beginning of profound healing. Because for the first time, she wasn't alone with it anymore.

My inner child closed her eyes and opened the door to her childhood. Slowly, she stepped back into a world she hadn't visited in years. When she reopened her eyes, she found herself inside her old home, surrounded by the familiar presence of her parents and sister. Everything looked just as she remembered it. Her mother stood in the kitchen, cooking - the same way she used to during those long-ago evenings. She looked exactly as she had been etched in her childhood memories: her green eyes shining gently beneath a matching green headband, the colour a striking contrast against the warm, dark tone of her skin. Her mother smiled softly, reminding her of the things that needed to be done before dinner, just like she used to. Without saying a word, my inner child stepped forward and wrapped her arms around her mother in a long, silent hug - a gesture filled with longing, grief, and the quiet hope of reconnection. She wanted to stay there forever, nestled close to her mother's chest, listening to the steady rhythm of her heartbeat and feeling the comforting warmth of her embrace. At that moment, time dissolved. There were no words - only the deep, unspoken knowing that they had both missed each other. The hug held everything: grief, longing, love, and the silent ache of what was never said.

Then, her eyes moved to the living room. Her father sat on the couch, watching television, just as he used to. From the beginning of this journey into her past, she had no difficulty recognizing the coldness that had always surrounded him. It was familiar - painfully so. He didn't turn his head. He may not have even noticed she was there. That absence, that silence, had long been a part of her story. And even in this inner return, nothing had changed.

Her heart began to race as she walked toward her bedroom, the room where she had spent the first fourteen years of her life. With each step, decades of grief and longing stirred within her. She had dreamed of opening that door again for so long that her heart felt as if it might leap from her chest. Slowly, she turned the handle and stepped inside. Everything was still there. Her bed, unchanged. Her desk, familiar - but this time, it sat empty. No books to read, no homework to finish. Just stillness. And for the first time, she was truly present in the space where so much of her story had begun. All she wanted was to lie down on her bed and gaze once more at the familiar walls of her room - the place that, long ago, had offered her a sense of safety. Just being there, in that stillness, felt like a quiet return to a part of herself she had almost forgotten.

As she made her way back to the kitchen, the sound of laughter caught her attention. It was her father's voice, loud and animated. He was surrounded by a small group of people, telling jokes that didn't seem to land well. Even though she was still too young to understand the word "misogyny," she could feel it in the air. She noticed the discomfort in the faces around him; how their smiles were forced, their laughter strained. Yet her father kept going, seemingly oblivious or unconcerned with how others perceived him. Then, he shifted to giving advice on how to lose weight, speaking with the same confident tone as if he were an authority on the subject. Her mother stepped in, cutting through the moment with biting words that humiliated him in front of everyone. She called out his hypocrisy, pointing out his struggles with weight, exposing the hollowness of his advice. The room went silent. And once again, the young girl witnessed a familiar dynamic - a moment charged with shame, disconnection, and the unspoken wounds that shaped her home.

As she stood there, silently observing the scene, her little heart swelled with confusion and discomfort. She didn't have the words to name what she felt, but her body remembered: the tension in her shoulders, the unease in her stomach, the sharp sting of secondhand shame. She didn't know why it felt wrong; just that it did. She couldn't understand why her father seemed so detached from the feelings of others, or why her mother's sharp response, though truthful, still left the air heavy with humiliation.

At that moment, her inner child didn't know where to stand. She didn't know who to trust. The people who were supposed to guide and protect her were tangled in their own unresolved pain, and all she could do was watch. She felt invisible. Small. Like her presence didn't matter. Again, she told herself that it didn't matter. The moment wasn't about being seen, it was about seeing.

Though, her Self stepped in. Tooted, calm, and compassionate, her Self assured her that she didn't have to carry that confusion alone. Her protective parts, once burdened with the job of keeping these memories locked away, now recognized that she no longer had to make sense of this chaos on her own. The Self gently stepped forward, kneeled beside her, and reminded her: *"You didn't imagine that discomfort. You felt what was real. You were wise, even then. You didn't deserve to feel invisible. Your voice, your emotions, your presence - they matter deeply."*

And at that moment, the little girl began to exhale. For the first time, she felt seen. Not by her father. Not even by her mother. But by the most important witness of all - her own Self.

I only wanted skies to chase,
Bare feet, wild dreams, a boundless place.
To laugh without the weight of why,
To touch the stars, to climb the sky.

They told me "Grow," but not "Be free,"
They gave me rules, not wings or sea.
So I became a careful child,
Quiet heart, emotions filed.

My mirror shows a stranger's face,
Years I can't replace or trace.
I watch my life like passing rain,
Half in longing, half in pain.

> I miss the wind, I miss the sun,
> The me I was when life was fun.
> Before the masks, before the fear,
> Before I learned to disappear.
>
> The world was once a place to play,
> Not just survive or shrink away.
> Now time moves fast, and I feel slow
> A guest within my own shadow.
>
> Yet still I hear my younger voice,
> A whisper lost beneath the noise.
> "Come back," she says, "we're not yet done,
> There's still a place beneath the sun."

After peeling off the layers of time, my inner child acknowledged that her father was emotionally unavailable and passive; a man who appeared to be dominated by my mother, lacking a strong will of his own. During her childhood, she could only perceive her father through the lens of her mother, who constantly highlighted his shortcomings and insecurities. Her mother's voice became the filter through which she understood him. But as she grew older and more attuned to her own perceptions, she began to see a different truth. Beneath his passivity, her father had been quietly pulling the right strings to serve his own interests. He was not merely weak or insecure, but calculated in his own subtle way. He presented himself as a neglectful, self-absorbed person; a man consistently centered on his own comfort and ease. Relationships, to him, were not sacred or reciprocal. People became tools, conveniences to be used when needed and discarded when not.

This realization brought clarity to the confusion that once clouded her. It helped her see that both parents, in their own ways, had contributed to the emotional landscape she had grown up in. The child who once sought affection and understanding from a distant father could now grieve what she didn't receive; not with blame, but with truth. And in that truth, her healing found deeper roots.

My inner child couldn't recall having an interesting conversation with her father or getting a hug from him, unless she asked for one. Although she spoke with him countless times, their conversations were always very much the same, casual and monotone, around issues that were pressing in the moment. She always had the feeling that she never truly got to know who her father was, because all she could see was a shell; a man imprisoned in his own mind, unable to connect emotionally. Unlike many self-absorbed individuals who at least develop cognitive empathy, he showed no desire to understand others or place himself in their shoes. He seemed incapable of emotional resonance. The only responsibilities he acknowledged as a parent were to "*put food on the table*" and provide "*a roof over our heads.*"

In his eyes, that alone defined good parenting. His standard was based solely on what he had received from his own parents, and he saw no reason to go beyond that. He never questioned whether his children needed more or different forms of care. He was a man who measured love by duty and provision, not by presence or connection. And for my inner child, that absence left a deep and quiet ache; a longing not just for a father, but for a connection that never had the chance to take root.

Reflecting on these memories revealed the void her father had left in her life. My inner child longed to be close to him, feel protected and learn from his wisdom. But over time, she was forced to accept his distance, even though his emotional inaccessibility never truly made sense. His absence cast a long shadow, shaping her choices in subtle, unconscious ways. As she sought safety in others, she ended up gravitating toward people who mirrored his detachment.

As she continued to unpack her childhood memories, my inner child turned toward her relationship with her mother, her hero, her anchor, the person she loved most. To her, her mother was perfect, and being close to her felt like everything she ever needed. Sensitive and deeply attuned, my inner child craved her mother's love and attention. She worked hard to meet every expectation, doing all she could to avoid causing her even the slightest disappointment.

My inner child will never forget the nights when her mother shared stories from her own childhood. Those stories transported her to a distant, unfamiliar time; a space that felt cold and unsafe. Still, she listened intently, absorbing every word, trying to understand her mother's pain and experiences. Her mother was born just a year after the Second World War ended; a time scarred by economic hardship, social upheaval, and the lingering wounds of trauma. When she was only three months old, her parents separated. Both would go on to remarry and have more children, but neither remained in her life. She was raised by her maternal grandmother, and it was only in that small, humble home that she felt truly loved and protected.

Occasionally, she visited her birth mother, who was often too overwhelmed with other children to pay much attention. Her father died when she was still very young, so she never had the chance to know him. In the midst of poverty and emotional abandonment, it was her grandmother who became her world. Despite the heavy burden of her time, her grandmother gave everything she could, especially during those first nine years, when she was the only one who cared for her. Her only companion during those years was a cat, her little partner in mischief. Together, they'd sneak into cupboards and steal treats meant to be saved for later, a small rebellion that brought joy in an otherwise heavy childhood.

Still, the fear of abandonment took root early. Even her grandmother's love couldn't fully soothe the wound left by her parents' absence. Deep down, she carried resentment toward her mother for leaving her behind. And just as she was beginning to feel some stability, more emotional damage was done. Her aunt offered to take her to the city and enroll her in school, but only on the condition that she babysit her cousin. Even the offer of care came with a price.

My inner child felt deeply connected to her mother's sorrow. Her heart broke when she saw her cry, confessing that the only person who had ever truly loved her was her grandmother. In those moments, my inner child felt overwhelming gratitude for having her mother present in her life every day, and for the opportunity to receive her love.

Because of her deep abandonment wounds, her mother struggled to believe she was lovable. She often felt unworthy and had difficulty regulating her emotions. Much of her focus was directed outward: on other people's behaviour, the injustices she faced, and the disappointments life had dealt her.

As a tailor, she had a wide social network, but her relationships were often strained. She found it difficult to set healthy boundaries and frequently overshared her pain: with neighbours, clients, and even us, her children. It wasn't malice; it was her inner child, still aching for the attention and validation she never received. She constantly searched outside of herself for reassurance, trying to feel seen, heard, and safe.

Though her mother expressed affection, she often seemed lost in her own world, consumed by unresolved pain. Her sorrow, constant complaints, and frequent irritability became part of the emotional backdrop of our daily lives. Even before her health began to decline, before Alzheimer's gradually took her away, she often behaved in childlike ways: seeking constant reassurance, questioning whether my inner child truly loved her, and needing proof that she still mattered.

Sometimes my inner child still wondered whether the affection she received from her mother came from genuine care or from her own need to be seen, loved, and mirrored. Perhaps it was both. She did show her affection, especially when she was very young, but then it often felt like she was comforting her mother more than the other way around. Once my inner child started to grow up, she noticed how her mother reacted with jealousy, resenting the time she spent caring for herself or nurturing relationships outside of her. Her mother would say she felt replaced. It didn't feel like unconditional love to my inner child. It felt like love wrapped in need, love that demanded rather than offered space to grow.

Now that I am an adult, I understand something I couldn't fully grasp as a child: that true parental love is given freely. Parents are meant to make sacrifices out of love, not to bind their children with unspoken debts, nor to expect them to repay that love by sacrificing their own adult lives. Healthy parental love is unwavering, spacious, and emotionally attuned. It offers the child a secure foundation from which to explore the world and develop a sense of self that is both autonomous and connected. It does not demand perfection or total obedience to earn affection. Instead, it welcomes the child as they are, curious, flawed, and unique, and meets their emotional needs. In this kind of love, a parent is a steady presence. Healthy love encourages open dialogue, mutual respect, and emotional safety. It doesn't shame or manipulate; it guides, protects, and nurtures. Most importantly, it allows the child to feel safe enough to make mistakes and express emotions.

Decades have passed, yet my inner child still feels the sting of her mother's words. Her mother compared her children, using labels like "*smart*" and "*stupid*," measuring them by their ability to earn good grades effortlessly. Her words cut deep, leaving lasting scars that quietly eroded my inner child's self-esteem and confidence for many years. She saw her children as extensions of herself and measured their adaptability, referring to their ability to go with the flow without needing constant attention. After my inner child was born, her mother decided to stay home to care for her because my inner child was frequently ill as a baby and had no one else to support her. Years later, her mother often reminded my inner child of the sacrifices she had made for her - using them, at times, as leverage to get what she expected in return. If she didn't do certain things for her mother, she would accuse her of not truly loving her.

My inner child struggled to face the full truth about her mother. She could see the wounded child inside her; the part still frozen in the pain of abandonment, desperately seeking happiness through others. She also saw the functional part of her mother, the one who managed daily responsibilities, kept the house running, and cared for us in practical ways. But what was hardest to admit was that her mother also had protective parts that used guilt, manipulation, and emotional pressure to get her inner child's needs met. These parts, though likely born from her own inner child's suffering, often caused harm. And my inner child was one of the people who felt that pain.

While her mother's inner child did care for her children, perhaps seeing reflections of herself in her children, her protective parts were deeply judgmental. Instead of taking steps to change the course of her life, she often placed blame on others: her husband, her children, anyone but herself. Not only did she treat her children unequally, but she also manipulated, gaslighted, and projected her insecurities onto them, as if they were merely extensions of her, rather than individuals with their own needs and identities. Her mother carried a deep sense of alienation throughout her life. She was haunted by the fear of rejection, battled persistent feelings of worthlessness, and struggled with insecurity in nearly all her relationships. Her constant need for reassurance was a cry from the child inside her, a child who never truly felt safe, seen, or loved unconditionally.

My inner child struggled to acknowledge just how hurtful many of her mother's actions were, how deeply they wounded her self-esteem and distorted her understanding of love. It wasn't until early adolescence that she allowed herself to see the truth:

her mother was not as loving as she had once believed.

Around that time, a new protector began to emerge, one who dared to give voice to the pain my inner child had long silenced. Still, her voice wasn't strong. Even as my inner child felt hurt by her mother's behaviours, she clung desperately to the idealized image she had initially created. The guilt ran deep. Over the years, the perfect image of her mother began to crumble, slowly, piece by piece. But it wasn't until she began writing this memoir that she fully confronted the painful truth: her mother had long embodied the traits of a vulnerable, self-absorbed person.

Reflecting on the past helped my inner child begin to make sense of the confusion she had always felt around her mother's behaviour. At times, her mother spoke with a soft, gentle voice, seeking love, attention, and validation to soothe her own wounded inner child. At other times, she became overbearing and demanding, insisting on total obedience and lamenting that she was not respected. This emotional inconsistency left my inner child yearning for stability, consistency, and emotional safety in her relationships. Yet some of her protective parts often ignored the red flags that contradicted what she longed to find, because hearing overbearing, demanding, and critical voices felt familiar to them. My inner child longed deeply for love, but her protectors could not recognize that the reality before them did not bring the feeling they were searching for.

My Self now understands that my parents were deeply co-dependent and profoundly unhappy together. My father spent most of his life in the army, while my mother stayed home to raise us. As a tailor, she worked from home, a profession she loved and in which she was respected. But because it wasn't a registered business, she had no pension or financial independence in the last years of her life. Relying on my father during times when she had no clients was difficult for her. He resented sharing money and demanded to know how every cent was spent. In many ways, my mother gave me my first lessons in feminism. She spoke out loudly against patriarchy and control, and she often criticized my father's misogynistic behavior. Yet, she continued living with him, even after he crossed a line no partner ever should.

He raised his hands against her once. Just once, but once was enough. I was only a few years old, and it became the first traumatic memory of my life. I still remember the moment vividly: my mother's scream cutting through the air, her voice filled with fear and fury: *"Get away from me! Leave me alone! Don't you ever touch me again!"* That image never left me. It imprinted itself in my body, marking the beginning of my awareness that something was terribly wrong.

My inner child never witnessed kindness between my parents; no gestures of affection, no words that conveyed love. On the contrary, they seemed to go out of their way to express their unhappiness. Their marriage resembled more of a contract, a pact to endure each other until the end, rather than a bond built on love or mutual respect. Their daily interactions reflected the weight of that commitment more than any emotional connection.

Years later, my inner child learned a truth that had long been hidden: her father had cheated on her mother with her best friend. For a long time, her inner child couldn't bear to face it. She clung to denial, unable to accept the betrayal. Only recently has she begun to see things more clearly, recognizing in both parents the patterns and pathologies of self-absorbed behaviour.

Until the end of her mother's life, her parents seemed to bring out the worst in each other. The only time they functioned as a team was when they turned against others. They would zero in on the smallest perceived slight, fuel each other's complaints, and insist they were being mistreated. In those moments, united in bitterness, they finally acted like partners. But their unity came from shared resentment, not love.

When my inner child was fourteen, her mother decided to leave our apartment in the city and move to the countryside. She longed for freedom and a house with open space, a home on the ground. To support her decision, she framed it as an act of care. She said it was for my inner child's benefit, that she was "*too reliant on her,*" and needed to become more independent. But for my inner child, it was the first time she felt discarded. Her mother left and she didn't come back. Once she settled into her new life, it was as if my inner child no longer existed in the same way. And then, eventually, her father followed her. At first, he tried to keep one foot in both worlds, commuting between the city and the countryside. But after his retirement, he too disappeared from my inner child's daily life. She was discarded, first by her mother, then by her father.

From the moment she moved into her new home, her mother no longer seemed concerned about my inner child's basic needs, essential things such as food, clothing. She was also not concerned about my inner child's dreams related to her future. In her mother's eyes, my inner child's chances of achieving independence or higher education seemed not just unlikely, but impossible, because she was her *"stupid"* child. So, it quickly became clear to my inner child that she would have to rely on herself.

The unseen child missed her mother so deeply that she would leave school early on Fridays just to catch the bus that would take her to her. Despite the pain of abandonment, my inner child never stopped loving her parents. She was pure, tender-hearted, and so eager to be loved that she felt guilty even for questioning the kind of love they gave her.

During my inner child's early teenage years, another protective part began to emerge: a part that tried to help my inner child cope with the pain of being unseen. This part pushed back against the scars left by my inner child's mother's harsh words and believed, however quietly, that she deserved more. But the battle wasn't easy. She, too, was young and still learning what life was about.

Our core beliefs are formed in early childhood, etched deeply into our minds, shaping how we see ourselves and the world. My inner child and the protective parts that grew around her made sense of our experiences through the narrow lens of what they knew, limited by youth, shaped by pain. Many of those beliefs only grew stronger over time. Every time my inner child's voice was silenced, whether through criticism, neglect, or guilt, it reinforced the message that she was invisible. And so the cycle continued.

The first traumatic experiences of my inner child were caused by the very people she loved the most. Her early life was a patchwork of moments, some filled with warmth, others overshadowed by her parents' inability to manage their own emotions. She never truly experienced unconditional love, because her parents themselves didn't know what real love looked or felt like. Their absence, whether physical or emotional, their invalidation, and the verbal and emotional abuse she endured slowly eroded her sense of self-worth. She began to believe, deep down, that she wasn't good enough. That she wasn't lovable.

Ancestral trauma. The deep-rooted issues stemming from my family's unhealed past traumas created the cognitive dissonance that I have experienced since then. My inner child internalized the emotional and psychological patterns passed on by her parents and shaped her destiny. The internal conflict that I've experienced throughout my life was caused by the opposing views of my parts, as some of my protective parts have tried to build resiliency without creating and fostering a unified approach in supporting my inner child. While my inner child was naive, thinking that all people had good intentions, a protective part of me saw people's true actions; my inner child saw herself as a victim, thinking that she couldn't overcome the obstacles from her life by herself, while a part of me wanted more for her life than her parents wished for her; my inner child felt invisible, while a part of me wanted to be recognized and have her voice heard.

As I carried with me the legacy of my parents' traumas, my healing required radical acceptance and understanding of human limitations.

> She never left,
> just sat so still
> beneath the noise,
> behind the will.
>
> A glance, a breath,
> and there she shone
> not lost, not hurt,
> just never alone.

Chapter 3

The New Me

> I rise with quiet strength,
> no longer bound by old chains.
> My heart holds both scars and light,
> my spirit walks freely,
> claiming joy, love, and peace as mine.

The truth about the root cause of my struggles became clear more than thirty years later, when I finally saw it. A moment that felt like yet another setback revealed itself to be a powerful catalyst - an invitation to slow down, reflect, and make peace with my past so I could create a more authentic and fulfilling future. My pain became fertile ground for growth. It illuminated the path toward healing, showing me that beneath the suffering was an opportunity for profound transformation.

I found the courage to confront my internal world, bravely and honestly. I welcomed the voices of all my parts and allowed them to share their unfiltered truths, stories they had carried for years in silence. Each part deserved to be heard. Each one had protected my inner child in the only ways they knew how. Only when they embarked on this journey of introspection together did they realize how much they needed one another. Through connection, understanding, and compassion, they began to transform. Healing didn't come from silencing the pain, it came from listening to it with love.

In the past, I kept my heart open to everyone and I gave people access to the most tender parts of me, even when they didn't deserve it. In doing so, I allowed others to hurt me. Abuse from self-absorbed people leaves deep wounds. It leads many to isolation, anxiety, depression, and sometimes even post-traumatic stress. It shatters self-worth, erodes confidence, and undermines the ability to trust, not just others, but ourselves. It can also steal the belief that life can be better. In response, many survivors learn to protect themselves by shutting down. They close their hearts, hide their pain, and remain silent to avoid further harm. But I have chosen a different path.

Rather than keeping my story locked away, I want to share it. I don't share it to seek validation, as I know who I am, and I hold that truth firmly within me. I don't need approval, and hurtful comments; if they come, will not define me. They speak only of the speaker, not of me. The vulnerability I embrace by telling my story is an act of self-love. And it's a gift for anyone who sees themselves in my words, for those who are searching for hope and are ready to begin their own journey toward healing.

Like most people, I used to run from pain. But this time, I learned that the only way out was through. I turned inward, disconnecting from the outside world as much as I could. In the silence of my home, I allowed myself to feel everything, no matter how painful, no matter who caused it. I accepted that some people chose to hurt me, repeatedly and intentionally. But I also took responsibility for the choices I made, or the choices made by some of my parts.

At first, I was frozen in pain. But little by little, I began to understand the internal battle I had been carrying for so long. There were moments when the weight of it all felt unbearable, like I was experiencing the full accumulation of every wound I'd ever buried. Some old hurts resurfaced, raw and vivid, as if no time had passed at all. And still, I stayed with it.

I remember feeling shame a few times as a child, but nothing compared to what I felt then. This time, it was suffocating. It felt like I was submerged underwater, unable to breathe. And for months, that feeling wouldn't go away. As I looked back on all the disappointments I had carried throughout my life, I couldn't understand why I had allowed so many people to hurt me, again and again. At first, it seemed as if those people weren't the only ones who had caused harm, but some of my own protective parts had become unwitting participants. They were supposed to protect my inner child. Instead, they had let her down. These parts blamed themselves for the pain she endured, especially each time they forgave those who hurt her, hoping things would be different.

But the cycle repeated. And each time it did, my inner child was left more wounded, more confused, and more alone.

In the beginning, identifying my parts was difficult. Each time I tried to connect with them, I could feel their pain - and it was overwhelming. They had protected my inner child like an invisible armor, shielding her from revisiting the memories she had buried and from fully understanding the ripple effect her childhood had cast across her life.

The trauma of being emotionally abandoned by her parents shaped how she sought love, respect, and stability. She looked for those things in others, often settling for far less than she deserved. My protective parts carried that pain too. They did what they could to help her survive, even if it meant avoiding the truth. Often, they needed breaks. This process wasn't linear. But slowly, as I wrote this memoir and gave each part the space to speak, they began to relax. Each step forward brought a sense of relief, a quiet reassurance that they no longer had to carry the burden alone.

When they finally understood the purpose of this work, everything began to shift. They not only acknowledged the need to adapt their skill sets to better protect my inner child's well-being, but they also let go of the fear of being judged and criticized, a fear that had once paralyzed them. My Self welcomed each of them with compassion, inviting them to speak freely about their experiences, intentions, perspectives, and hopes for the future.

This process of introspection softened the weight of their past. It brought a growing sense of calm, moment by moment, and slowly built their resilience. In learning to understand themselves and one another, they began to heal, not through control or suppression, but through connection and shared purpose.

The desire to do this work became a powerful force within me. Spending time alone with my thoughts didn't feel difficult, it felt necessary, even sacred. It became a daily practice, more meaningful than anything else during that period. My inner child and protective parts no longer wished to avoid the past or remain disconnected from one another. Instead, they found the courage to open up, to share, and to learn together. They made a conscious commitment to offer themselves what they had once so freely given to others: kindness, understanding, love, flexibility, and compassion.

> I step into the morning unafraid,
> shedding the shadows that clung too long.
> The weight of old voices,
> the chains of expectation,
> fall quietly behind me,
> and I breathe in a life of my own design.
>
> I carry the echoes of my inner child,
> her laughter, her wonder, her quiet tears,

and honor them with each deliberate step.
No longer silenced by fear,
no longer shrinking to fit the world,
I stretch into the fullness of being.

My hands build, my heart opens,
my mind listens to the rhythm of my soul.
Joy is no longer a distant guest;
it dances beside me,
tender, luminous, insistent.

I love with clarity,
choose with courage,
forgive with grace.
The past whispers, but it no longer rules
its lessons shape me,
but do not define me.

I am whole.
I am fierce.
I am free.
I am the keeper of my own story,
and in this becoming,
I am finally home.

3.1 Healing My Inner Child

*A hand to hold,
a gaze that sees,
a heart that answers
silent pleas.*

*A soft "you matter,"
just because
no need to earn,
no fear, no fuss.*

*A steady light,
both kind and true
the love you needed,
just for you.*

The emotional injuries of our childhood don't dissipate over time. Until she began her healing journey, my inner child remained frozen in time, stuck at the moment when her parents left to build their new home. For her, nothing mattered more than having a family and stability. Sadly, the repeated painful experiences of her childhood slowly chipped away at her belief that she was lovable. She carried the emotional scars of her ancestors, unspoken wounds that shaped the inner story she told herself about who she was and how she was meant to be, particularly in her relationships with others. My inner child longed to be loved, accepted, and safe, firmly believing that every person is worthy of love, but instead, she was ridiculed for being different. They called her *"too sensitive," "a dreamer," "stupid,"* and *"naive."* Over time, she was forced to come to terms with a painful truth: the people she needed the most were emotionally unavailable and dismissive of her very essence.

Before she began to heal, my inner child opened her heart without hesitation, unable to recognize people's true intentions. She believed that everyone was as loving and genuine as she was. For most of her life, she searched for kindness in people's words, trusting that what they said reflected the goodness in their souls. She focused on the good she saw in others, often overlooking the red flags in their behaviour. She could see their potential, and even when she was hurt, she stayed, refusing to think less of them.

Although she is certain that healthy relationships are based on good communication, honesty about one's intentions, desires, fears, insecurities, and commitment to learn and support, respect, and love, over the years, my inner child gradually adjusted to relationships that didn't always reflect these principles. While struggling to camouflage her disappointments, my inner child forgot how to smile, as she carried the weight of her unspoken trauma. She was too tired to cry and too scared to make a change. She was just surviving, wanting something outside of her to change. Therefore, to heal, she had to remove the bandages she had applied to her wounds over the years and leave them open to heal properly.

As she began to revisit her childhood memories, my inner child found herself constantly thinking about the people she had loved the most. Her thoughts kept the energetic ties between them alive, tethering her to the past. She became caught in a cycle of painful rumination, repeatedly asking herself, *"Why was I born into this family?"* Over time, she came to a quiet, yet powerful realization - this wasn't her choice. It took time for her to discern reality from illusion. Moreover, she felt energetically connected to some of the people from her past. Often, she would wake abruptly from dreams in which they appeared, speaking to her as if trying to reach her. She felt an intense pull toward them, searching for answers to her inner questions.

As part of her healing, my inner child had to confront the reality of her relationships with her family and other people from her past. It was no longer an option to bury her head in the sand to avoid seeing the truth. She had to fully acknowledge that continued contact with those who had chosen to hurt her would only reopen old wounds. Establishing a firm "no contact" boundary became essential as a protective measure to prevent further harm and allow space for reflection on the patterns of behaviour that had caused her so much pain.

Solitude became sacred in her healing journey. It offered the quiet she needed to disentangle herself from the emotional cords still tying her to the people who had once felt familiar. In that stillness, she could begin to dismantle the illusions they had projected onto her and rediscover who she truly was, apart from their influence. She came to value the protective gates she built around herself, not as walls to isolate, but as boundaries to honour her peace. In this space, distractions had no place; only healing was welcome.

My Self gently held space for her pain and reminded her that the answers she sought were already within. Gradually, through deep introspection and reflection on her past, she uncovered the truths she had long been seeking. With each memory, especially the fleeting shifts in their facial expressions that exposed their inner conflicts and the emotional armour shielding their own wounded inner child, she began to see things clearly. She recognized how they had mirrored her light, drawn to her energy in an unconscious attempt to avoid confronting their reflection. They crafted personas to shape how they wanted to be perceived, illusions designed to hide their unresolved pain.

When she questioned herself and doubted her perceptions, she didn't retreat. Instead, she stood firm and resisted the powerful urge to reach out to those she once believed had loved her. Missing them felt like missing a part of herself, and holding back from calling them was like fighting against her own instincts. But each time temptation crept in, her protective parts gently stepped in, reminding her of the pain these people had caused. They helped her hold onto the truth: that she could not allow those who had hurt her to regain power over her life.

Her Self stood beside her with quiet strength, cautioning her that reconnecting would only lead to more confusion and heartache. But the warnings came not as harsh commands, but as acts of care - soft, steady reassurances that she was being looked after, and that choosing herself was not selfish, but necessary. My inner child was never truly alone; she was part of a sisterhood. In moments of doubt, she turned to the other parts of herself, those who carried less emotional attachment to the people from her past. Through their clearer eyes, she was able to reexamine her experiences and see them for what they truly were.

It was painful to accept the truth: that none of these people truly understood love. To them, love meant the complete abandonment of oneself in service to their needs. It was as if they expected her to drink a cup of poison each day, smile through the pain, and offer words of affection just to soothe their fragile inner child. What they called love was, in reality, control wrapped in sweet words. In moments of intense pain, my inner child wished she could stop loving these people, but that proved difficult. Then she remembered: she had never loved their shadow parts, the aspects of them that inflicted harm. What she loved was their inner child, the part of them who, like her, had once longed for love, safety, and belonging.

By stepping into their shoes and viewing their struggles through a trauma-informed lens, she came to understand that their inner child had endured similar wounds. Like her, they wrestled with the belief that they were unlovable. Like her, they craved connection and acceptance. For my inner child, love was never fleeting or conditional; it was real and enduring. Her mistake wasn't in loving their inner child. It was in overlooking their shadow parts and denying the real impact of their harmful actions on her.

While reviewing her memories with these people, my inner child realized that she had attached to these people because of the stories she had created in her mind around them.

My inner child's attachment to her parents was both a biological instinct and an emotional lifeline, woven into her from birth. Like all children, she loved them without conditions, without tallying harm against kindness. That love was as natural as breathing, rooted in the belief that they were her protectors, her safe place in the world, even when reality did not always match that hope. Despite their flaws, they had given her life and, in those early years, provided for her needs: nutritious meals, clean clothes, and a room full of toys. Her mother wasn't always distant or cruel; there were moments of care and gentleness that she held onto fiercely, magnifying them in her heart to sustain her through the harder days.

That unconditional love became the soil where her protective stories grew. As children, we often see what we want to see, especially when our sense of safety depends on it. Whenever hurtful moments surfaced, she instinctively reshaped them into something more bearable, her mind smoothing sharp edges and filling in gaps with imagined warmth. A missed hug became a sign of busyness, not rejection. A harsh word became an attempt at guidance. These stories were not lies to her; they were lifelines, bridges that kept her tethered to the hope that her parents loved her in the way she needed. In holding onto these narratives, she preserved her sense of belonging, even when the reality was far more complicated.

Reflecting on her mother's difficult childhood and comparing her experience to the hardships many other children faced at the time, she often felt lucky to have her parents in her life. She didn't yet understand the complexity of her parents' struggles, particularly the impact of unaddressed mental health issues. But she clung to that early, comforting image of her parents and was unwilling to let it go. That was her family, and she loved them. Even as the cracks in that image began to show, she didn't question them; instead, she questioned herself. She believed the fault must lie within her.

As a child, her sense of self was shaped by how others treated her and what they said about her. When her mother called her "*stupid*," she absorbed that message as truth. Her worth was tied to her academic performance, and because not all of her grades were A+, she was seen - and began to see herself - as not smart enough. If she wasn't intelligent enough, then she didn't believe in her opinions and ability to make her own decisions.

When our childhood wounds remain unhealed, we often find ourselves trapped in confusion, unconsciously drawn to people who reflect those very wounds back to us. We mistake familiarity for love, falling in love not with who someone truly is, but with the dream of what we've always longed for. From the early moments of a connection, we begin projecting an idealized image onto them, one shaped by our unmet needs and the hope of rewriting our past. Often, this image is a reflection of the parent who couldn't give our inner child the unconditional love it needed. My inner child followed that same path, unknowingly participating in the illusion she helped create, reinforcing the distorted reality she lived within.

Her Self gently encouraged her to begin emotionally detaching from those who had hurt her, not by pretending they didn't exist, but by consciously choosing not to dwell on them. This wasn't easy. They still lived in her heart, and her mind often refused to let them go. Some days, she succeeded; on others, she did not. Her progress was slow but steady. In time, she came to understand that grieving those relationships was a necessary step. Only by fully mourning what she had lost-or perhaps never truly had-could she begin to sever the emotional ties. In doing so, she let go of their emotions and finally began reconnecting with her own.

At the beginning of her healing journey, my inner child could only engage with her past on a cognitive level. A protective part within her had built an internal block, preventing her from expressing emotions, especially through tears. It was as if she stood atop a mountain of suppressed pain, unable to descend into the depths of it. But once that block was lifted, a profound emotional release followed. A single thought could now stir an avalanche of grief, sadness, and long-buried sorrow. Suddenly, crying became so accessible. She mourned not only the loss of her family but also the deep sense of safety and security that vanished when she lost her home. She grieved the years she had poured into people who never truly valued her. At times, it felt as though her heart was physically opening, accompanied by strange palpitations that seemed less like fear and more like pain finally leaving her body.

After several months of deep introspection and grieving, my inner child experienced a few brief kundalini awakenings. Each began with a distinct pressure at the base of her spine, just moments before a surge of emotion would flood through her, causing her entire body to shiver. She noticed sudden shifts in body temperature, waves of heat or chills that seemed to come from within. These experiences felt unsettling, almost overwhelming, especially because they left her so drained that she would fall into a deep, heavy sleep afterward. Yet, by the next day, the pressure in her spine would dissipate, and her mind would feel noticeably clearer, as though something had been released.

She didn't know how to name these experiences at first. It was only a few days later, guided by her Self, that she came across resources describing what she had gone through kundalini awakenings. These experiences became a profound reminder of the importance of embracing emotional pain rather than resisting it. Humans have not lost the innate ability to release fear and tension through the body - shaking, trembling, or crying, after deeply unsettling experiences. Whether this door opens depends not on the conscious mind alone, but on the subconscious's readiness to heal. When we begin to truly listen to the voice of the heart, the one yearning for self-love, we shine light into the hidden corners of our psyche, allowing the subconscious to begin releasing the pain it has carried for far too long.

This natural stress response is something many animals share - they instinctively shake off fear and tension after a threat. In contrast, most humans often disconnect from their bodies and emotions as a trauma response. In relationships with self-absorbed people, our nervous system enters survival mode - fight, flight, or freeze - dampening emotional pain to help us endure the experience. Over time, this protective state can become chronic, leaving us in a constant state of stress, hypervigilance, and emotional numbness. The tension that builds in our bodies often settles in the tailbone, which is energetically connected to the root chakra - the center tied to our sense of safety, survival, and belonging.

Healing is not just about reprocessing memories intellectually. It also requires a reconnection with the body. Crying is one of the most powerful ways to express and release deeply stored emotions. It allows the body to discharge the energetic residue of pain, making space for clarity, peace, and emotional freedom.

Those who are well-versed in kundalini awakening describe it as a process through which we shed mental conditioning and begin to experience deep inner peace and love. By then, my inner child had already come to understand that the love she needed would come from her internal system, but these experiences allowed her to *see* herself with newfound clarity. She embraced herself fully, limitations and strengths alike, recognizing her inherent right to be free, enough, and to no longer seek someone else to fill the void left by her parents' absence of love. Slowly but surely, the intensity of her emotions began to soften.

Gradually, it became easier for her to disconnect from those who had chosen to hurt her by shifting her focus inward. She made the conscious decision to offer herself the same care and devotion she had once given to others. She began treating herself with kindness, flexibility, commitment, awareness, stability, and hope for a better future. It would be dishonest to say that these changes came easily; they didn't. In some areas, she progressed quickly, staying focused and dedicated. In others, she struggled. The tendency to abandon herself lingered. But she didn't give up. Her protective parts offered gentle reminders of her goals and quietly encouraged her to keep going. Practices like Reiki, meditation, and writing this memoir helped her move forward. The Universe also responded - her Self softly whispered that an inverted mirror had been placed between her and the past, reflecting everything back for her to finally see with clarity.

It would be unrealistic to expect a life without sadness. The grief still lingers sometimes when she thinks of all that was lost. But instead of dwelling on the pain of her misfortunes, my inner child has come to honour her past. That past, with all its sorrow, became the lens through which she gained clarity: clarity that no one would ever again be allowed to take the peace she fought so hard to reclaim. She gave her pain meaning - it marked the beginning of her rebirth. True transformation doesn't arise from perfection, but from the courage to face life's hardships and grow beyond them. My inner child learned to release the limitations others had projected onto her and refused to be defined by them. She chose freedom, the freedom to create the life she had always longed for. She chose to be present in the now.

Throughout her life, my inner child was guided by the Universe through the presence of her Self. Even as a child, she could sense things before they happened at times, but once she began her healing journey, the signs from the Universe grew clearer and more frequent, reminding her that she was never alone, that she was intimately connected to everything around her. As she deepened her connection with her Self, her trust in this greater guidance returned. Doubt gave way to clarity. In her search to understand her past and find peace, she began receiving answers not only from within, through her protective parts, but also from sources outside of herself. A question that lingered at night was answered the next day. She would feel called to reach out to someone, only to discover that they held the exact insight she needed. Opportunities arrived precisely when she was ready for them. It was no longer a coincidence; it was alignment. And in that alignment, she found trust, healing, and the reassurance that she was always being supported.

My inner child was never truly alone. She never had been. Her Self was always there, whispering gently, offering guidance, patiently waiting for her to listen. In the past, she hadn't yet learned how to be receptive. But once her healing journey began, she discovered the power of stillness. All she needed to do was pause, turn inward, and trust. The voice of her Self became clear.

Knowing that the Universe saw her, *truly* saw her, brought a peace she had never known. She felt blessed in ways words could hardly express. In her darkest and most painful moments, it was the Universe, through her Self, that lit the path forward. She mattered. She always had. And now she finally understood that the Universe had always cared for her.

Her Self looked after her inner child carefully, bringing structure and consistency. Sleep and nourishment became priorities. Listening to quantum music and establishing a sleep routine brought immediate results. Rest became a cornerstone of her healing, giving her the energy to care for herself with compassion.

Each day, she felt a quiet pride in recognizing and meeting her own basic needs. If, in the past, she struggled to cook for herself when alone, reenacting the neglect from her childhood, now she made sure to eat nourishing meals throughout the day. It took time and practice to undo the ingrained patterns of self-abandonment. After her last kundalini awakening, she was intuitively guided to shift her diet. She gradually adopted a more intuitive way of eating, trusting her body's wisdom to support her healing.

She also began practicing mindfulness each night, grounding herself in the present and reconnecting with the Universe. Rumination, a common struggle for survivors of narcissistic abuse, began to quiet. No longer lost in looping thoughts and unhealed wounds, she began to focus on the now. Mindfulness improved her emotional regulation, sharpened her awareness, and replaced insomnia with the most restful sleep she'd ever known. Occasionally, a short mindful practice in the morning helped her step into the day with intention and clarity.

Through her Self, the Universe had guided her to discover the "resource spot" even before she trained in Brainspotting. During meditation, with eyes closed, she found this place, a deep well of safety and comfort. This was a powerful support tool for calming her nervous system and reducing hyperarousal, two key barriers to lead to a restful sleep. Though she had already experienced the quiet support of her Self, this realization amazed her. It was one more reminder that when body, mind, and spirit work in harmony, healing becomes not only possible but natural.

Knowing her Self and all her internal parts were there for her gave her inner child a profound sense of safety. Her needs were no longer invisible. She no longer had to search outside herself for someone to belong to, because she had found that sense of belonging within. Her unity with all parts of herself was enough. They had each other.

Finally, she understood the depth of Maya Angelou's words, when asked if she belonged to anyone:

"More and more... I belong to myself. I'm very proud of that. I am very concerned about how I look at Maya. I like Maya." (4)

As her protective parts began to heal, her inner child began to feel joy again, joy simply for being alive. She cherished waking up after a restful sleep, sipping her morning coffee while admiring the breathtaking view of the tiny city she now called home. She delighted in caring for her flowers, soaking in the peace that filled her days. As she found freedom from pain, her smile returned.

She twirls in sunlight, barefoot and free,
Chasing butterflies no one else can see.
Her laughter rings like a lullaby,
Painting joy across the sky.

She builds her castles out of sand,
Trusting waves, not fearing land.
With every giggle, every song,
She reminds me where I still belong.

Unburdened heart, so wild and mild
That's the magic of my inner child.
Alive, at peace, and full of grace
She's the light I now embrace.

3.2 Healing My "In Control" Protector

She came when trust broke,
when the ground no longer felt safe.
Not out of coldness
but devotion.

She built walls,
drew lines,
held the system steady
when the storm was too loud
to feel.

She silenced the past
so the child could function,
believing that stillness
was survival.

Logic was her language.
Order, her offering.
Feeling had no place
until the Self whispered,
there's more than one way to be strong.

She softened,
slowly.
Not by surrender,
but by listening.

Now, she protects healing.
Still vigilant.

But no longer afraid
of the heart.

There is a protective part of me who feels the deep need to stay in control. She emerged around the same time as my highly functioning part, and together, they make a strong team, working hand in hand to bring stability and build a secure future for my inner child. Her presence allows my highly functioning part to disconnect from external chaos and focus on her work. But at her core, this part was born from a breakdown of trust in others. Her primary role: to keep my inner child safe.

This "in control" part helped my inner child cope with painful childhood experiences by repressing some of her most difficult memories and emotions. After being discarded by her parents, my inner child often felt lonely, confused, and abandoned. There were even times when she lacked food because her parents had other priorities. The pain was overwhelming, so heavy that at moments, she became numb. It was in those moments that this part emerged, shielding her by suppressing unbearable emotions and memories, enabling her to function.

Years later, my inner child discovered that she couldn't recall many details from that period. While her memory was sharp in general, she had only vague impressions of those difficult years, and she was disturbed by her inability to piece them together. With conscious effort, she eventually retrieved some of them, only to find that the emotional intensity had faded. That's when she began to understand what this part had done for her, both the protection and the cost.

After the resurfacing of her unhealed wounds, my "in control" part wanted to move forward quickly. She still longed for something better, a life free from so much pain. She believed the way forward was to suppress those feelings again. To her, the choice seemed binary: either become a victim or fight. So she activated every survival instinct, pushing the entire system forward. But the more she forced progress, the more exhausted she became. Eventually, my Self intervened, urging her to slow down.

My highly functioning part gently introduced her to information about the healing power of crying, something she had previously rejected. But needing evidence, she sought scientific validation. She learned that crying activates the amygdala, which processes emotions, and the hypothalamus, which balances the sympathetic and parasympathetic nervous systems. Though, crying is not entirely an involuntary response influenced only by emotional factors, but a cognitive act too, governed by the prefrontal cortex, which allows us to decide when to express or suppress emotions. When crying, our body releases oxytocin and endorphins, easing both physical and emotional pain. Suppressing this natural emotional release can result in elevated cortisol levels, leading to immune dysfunction, anxiety, irritability, poor sleep, and emotional numbness. Crying is not a weakness. It is biology, healing, and self-love.

This understanding began to soften her. She slowly accepted that her role needed to evolve, not to push forward at all costs, but to allow room for feeling, release, and integration.

As her perspective shifted, she also became more willing to honour the needs of the inner child and other protective parts. She made space for solitude, not as an escape, but as a conscious act of self-care. She learned that time alone was not isolation, but nourishment.

Under the guidance of my Self, she also made the difficult yet necessary decision to go "no contact" with those who had harmed her inner child. This was not a weapon, like the silent treatment used by self-absorbed people; it was a boundary, a form of protection, and a declaration of her inner child's worth. There was no longer any desire to give kindness to people who had chipped away at the inner child's self-esteem. The door was closed, not out of bitterness, but clarity. These individuals did not love, honour, or protect her; they merely fed off external validation. That cycle had to end.

At first, this "no contact" approach was painful for her inner child, who had never drawn such firm boundaries before. But as healing began, she came to appreciate it. It became her shield, keeping out the energies that once drained her and giving her the space to reflect, observe life without becoming entangled in it. The actions of those who once hurt her provided all the evidence she needed to move forward without them. She found peace, not because they changed, but because she did.

Healing from abuse by self-absorbed individuals isn't a one-time event. It's an ongoing process, and one that takes constant tending. The boundaries that my "in control" part learned to establish are now non-negotiable. They're not just tools of survival - they are expressions of love for my inner child. They are standards and they are sacred.

One of her deepest vulnerabilities was the belief that she could only rely on herself. Even when the rest of the system acknowledged the guidance of the Universe through the Self, my "in control" part remained skeptical. She struggled to fully trust the unseen, believing in the kind of help that couldn't be measured or logically explained. To her, faith without empirical evidence felt unsafe.

Yet over time, she could no longer ignore the synchronicities - the quiet, almost imperceptible ways the Universe had protected and supported her inner child, sometimes in the final hour. She recalled moments at major crossroads when unseen forces had clearly intervened. She oscillated between doubt and belief, but kept searching, trying to weave these inexplicable experiences into a worldview that still made space for logic. Gradually, her skepticism began to soften, understanding that not everything unfolding around us can yet be scientifically explained. But that did not make it less real.

When she discovered the work of Robert Falconer, a pioneering therapist and international educator in Internal Family Systems therapy, who speaks openly about spirituality, spirit possessions, and guides, she felt a deep sense of ease. His work validated the experiences of her internal family system. She could now say with certainty: spirituality is indeed essential for healing trauma.

Although this protector has made important changes that benefit my internal system and seeing the growing strength and wisdom in my other protective parts, she still clings tightly to the reins. She has spent a lifetime scanning for danger, predicting outcomes, and building contingency plans, because to her, safety has always depended on being one step ahead. Even now, with evidence that my discernment is sharper and my boundaries stronger, she hesitates to let go. Trusting others feels like standing on a bridge without checking the weight limit first. She worries that if she loosens her grip, chaos will rush in and undo all we have worked for. Her vigilance is rooted not in mistrust of my abilities, but in the memory of a time when those abilities didn't exist, when mistakes were costly and betrayal was the rule, not the exception. She is learning slowly that her value is not in controlling every outcome, but in collaborating with the rest of my system to respond wisely when life unfolds beyond prediction.

I hold the reins with steady hand,
I map the rules, I make the plan.
Chaos knocks, I shut the door,
I've kept us safe, and so much more.

But sometimes strength becomes a wall,
And fear of falling blocks the call.
I long to rest, to trust, to feel
But loosening grip feels less than real.

3.3 Healing My Highly Functioning Protector

There is no shame
in pausing.

Even the tide rests
before returning.

Even the moon
lets go of fullness.

You do not
owe the world
constant blooming.

Let your breath soften.
let your heart
be held
by nothing at all.

Stillness is not
Laziness.

It is the soul
finding its shape
Again.

My inner child has always been protected by many parts, one of them being the highly functioning part. She is determined to give life meaning, create stability, and help fulfill the dreams that once felt impossible. Hardworking, mature, and deeply aware of her strengths, this part thrives on challenge. She's bold when needed, not for dominance, but for growth. Though she's learned to slow down and rest, it's never long before another goal ignites her spirit and she rises again, ready to expand her limits.

Unlike some protectors who take over, she doesn't like to dominate. Instead, she collaborates. She values every part of the internal system, knowing that healing comes from unity, not control.

This part emerged when my inner child was in high school and met her mentor, a kind and encouraging teacher who tutored her during a summer break. He offered not just guidance, but belief. He helped her realize my inner child wasn't "*stupid,*" as she'd been led to believe by her family. For the first time, she felt seen for her potential. Her tutor introduced her to the concept of *perseverance* and planted the seed of hope: that change was possible through consistent effort. That seed grew into my highly functioning part. This part found freedom through knowledge.

But the journey required more than persistence, it demanded inner reconciliation. From the beginning of her journey, my highly functioning part had to face a powerful inner critic, another protector, who believed safety meant staying small and unnoticed. This critic, forged in fear, urged caution and invisibility. Yet rather than silence or reject it, she chose collaboration. She asked the critic to trust her strength, to believe in the path she was carving. Eventually, a pact was formed. In doing so, she also gave the inner critic space to grow beyond inherited fears and limiting beliefs that never truly belonged to them.

Over time, she became the force that helped break the generational chains that once tried to reshape the inner child into someone she was never meant to be. Through unwavering dedication and love for her inner child, she became the first in her family to attend university, forging a new path where none had existed. Her journey, though marked by obstacles and detours, became an expression of that love: fierce, devoted, and unrelenting in its hope.

In university classrooms filled with unfamiliar voices and uncertain expectations, she persevered, carrying the silent hopes of generations before her. Beneath her steadfast drive lived the quiet chaos of undiagnosed ADHD: disorganization, overwhelm, and forgetfulness that had no name at the time. While others appeared to move through their days with ease, she struggled through invisible storms just to stay afloat. Deadlines became emotional minefields, lectures dissolved into static, and her self-worth swung between fleeting sparks of confidence and deep spirals of self-doubt.

Still, this protector pressed on because she had made a promise to her inner child: to build a life that felt like freedom. Quietly, the Self guided her toward resources that taught her how to organize her days. Alongside this, the "in control" protector stepped in to help her stay focused and grounded. Every assignment submitted, every exam passed, was more than academic achievement, it was a quiet revolution. With each small victory, she dismantled the unspoken ceilings that had once defined her lineage and offered her inner child a new reality rooted in choice, growth, and belonging.

What began as a pursuit of safety, dignity, and possibility gradually revealed a deeper motive: the unconscious longing to prove the inner child's worth to those who had never truly seen her. Each late-night study session became an offering, an act to affirm her value and rewrite the narrative she had inherited. For years, she forged ahead, unaware that she was still seeking validation from a presence that existed only in memory. It wasn't just ambition driving her; it was the quiet hope that someone might finally say she was enough. And when she finally recognized that the person she was trying to reach, her mother, no longer existed, something within her softened. She laid down her sword. The struggle, at last, had come to an end.

Her progress hasn't always been linear. Other protective parts, driven by fear or survival, often pulled in different directions. Their conflicting beliefs and behaviors drained her energy, slowed her progress, and tested her resolve. For a long time, she and the overgiving part were disconnected, each acting from separate wounds. When the overgiving part led the internal system, the highly functioning part's path was paused and diverted by other peoples' needs. Moreover, she often found herself pushing against forces far greater than her own internal drive. In the culture she was raised in, defined by patriarchy and rigid gender expectations, her ambition wasn't always welcomed, it was questioned, diminished, or quietly resented. A woman with dreams outside the home was often seen as unruly, self-centered, or ungrateful. She was taught, both directly and through unspoken rules, that her role was to support others, not to lead; to accommodate and sacrifice her own needs. Her desire to acquire more education and develop her career was often met with resistance, sometimes disguised as concern, other times as outright disapproval, or even sabotage. These cultural messages slowed her progress. Yet she never stopped. She kept studying and working, first in her home country, then after the move to Canada. Her core belief was simple but heavy: *the only way out is through hard work.*

That belief, though noble, came with burdens. Her relentless work ethic sometimes turned into over-functioning, especially when activated by other protectors. The risk-manager protector pushed for financial security, convinced that only through material stability could a safe future be built for the inner child. And so, the highly functioning part kept going. That pressure became overwhelming. Eventually, the toll became too great, mentally, physically, and emotionally. She had to face the cost of burnout and learn a new lesson: that a fulfilling life required balance.

As her healing began, she felt deep regret for the years lost to overwork. She recognized that proving her intellectual worth had once felt like the only way to gain value. But now, she began to understand that true self-worth doesn't come from academic accolades or overachievement; it comes from honouring the Self, from living in a way that includes joy and rest for her inner child. Though she cannot undo the choices of the past, my highly functioning part is now focused on a new mission: to bring joy into the inner child's life. While she made these realizations, all the other parts listened silently, bearing witness to the decades of effort, the endless striving, and the courage it took to keep going. No words could capture their gratitude.

Now, the healing energy of my Self radiates toward all protective parts. They no longer function in isolation or opposition. They are a team. The Self holds no judgment for how long healing has taken. After all, they've survived adversity since childhood. They deserved compassion, not demands for rapid transformation.

My highly functioning part is no longer just a protector; she is a builder, a restorer who now understands that life is not only about proving others wrong, but about living fully, gently, and joyfully.

After being abandoned by those who were meant to love and protect us, we don't immediately realize that we must learn to love ourselves. When we experience trauma early in life, our inner child often becomes frozen at that developmental stage, still searching, hoping for someone to rescue them and offer the love they never received. It can take years, sometimes even decades, to understand that no one will step into the role our caregivers were supposed to play. Parts of us may try to fill that role, but they often lack the wisdom and maturity needed to truly nurture. That wisdom is earned over time, and often only emerges after we've hit rock bottom, when looking outward no longer works, and we are forced to turn inward.

It is only then, when we begin to align with the values of our Self, that our protective parts can stop acting in opposition and start working in harmony. With this alignment, they can create the future they once believed was out of reach.

This understanding changed everything for my system. It helped my protective parts recognize one another's value and begin to commit, not just to survival or achievement, but to joy. They came together to create space for play, rest, and peace in our inner child's life. Because after all, life is not only about work. It's about living.

> Not every moment
> needs a sound.

Even the stars
shine
in silence.

Rest,
and let the light
find you.

3.4 Healing My Risk-Manager Protector

> She walked before storms
> with her eyes on the sky,
> reading the winds
> that others passed by.
>
> She built bridges in shadows
> before rivers could rise,
> and mapped out each turn
> with a steady, sharp mind.
>
> Not ruled by fear,
> but by vision and care,
> she guarded the path
> so we'd always get there.
>
> And when the road opened,
> clear, wide, and bright,
> she stepped to the side
> letting me take flight.

This part of me, the risk manager, was born the moment my inner child lost her family, home, and sense of stability. After her world fell apart, this part emerged to help her survive in a life marked by poverty and unpredictability. She learned to watch finances carefully and use every resource mindfully. Working closely with my highly functioning part, she focused on building a stable future for her inner child through education, employment, and consistent saving. To her, safety didn't mean luxury, but stability. Her motives were never rooted in jealousy or materialism; she simply wanted to ensure that the inner child would never again be unprotected.

Since this protective part came to life, she rarely allowed herself to fully relax, especially after we moved to Canada. As a first-generation immigrant, my highly functioning part carried the invisible burden of rebuilding from the ground up. Navigating unfamiliar systems, languages, and social expectations, she worked relentlessly to carve out a new beginning. But she didn't do it alone. The risk manager was always nearby, tracking risks, managing finances, and structuring each decision, hoping to bring her inner child closer to her dreams.

Yet, there were moments when this part's focus on safety was overshadowed by my overgiving part. Compelled by the inner child's longing for love and acceptance, the overgiving part would take the lead, prioritizing connection over stability. In those moments, the voice of the risk manager went quiet.

But the risk manager didn't collapse, she recalibrated. She had never feared being alone. On the contrary, she moved forward with even greater determination. She doubled down on budgeting, planning, and working toward the life she envisioned. Her drive had never been about fear, it was about never again depending on people who couldn't walk beside us with integrity.

After frequently reassessing priorities and often denying small comforts in favor of her desired security, she started noticing that enjoyment felt like a luxury she hadn't yet earned. Life became a delicate balance between survival and hope, between holding everything together and longing, quietly, for rest. Often prompted by the destroyer of ancestral trauma to pause and reflect, another protective part who worried that in her effort to protect, the risk-manager considered that she might be repeating the very behaviors she resented in her parents. Was she denying the inner child comfort and nourishment under the guise of safety? These questions unsettled her. She feared that, in protecting the child from instability, she had reinforced the belief that joy and rest were not deserved.

Some relief came through learning from Dr. Frank Anderson that we often internalize the fears and dysfunctions of our caregivers. This understanding helped her distinguish her motivations. The risk-manager protector didn't suffer when the overgiving part temporarily took the lead.

Still, she began to soften. She learned to expand the definition of safety, to include small joys, moments of rest, and the acknowledgment that the inner child deserved more than just survival. Eventually, she had to confront a painful truth: she may never be able to fulfill every dream the inner child held. But she also recognized that chasing those dreams at all costs could mean missing what was already within reach: connection, presence, and peace. Healing, for her, became the art of recalibrating, not abandoning her mission, but revising it.

>She didn't long for diamonds,
>nor reach for the skies -
>just needed a moment
>to silence the cries.
>
>She folded her dreams
>in the corners of time,
>and walked through the years
>like a soft, steady rhyme.
>
>But now she sits quietly
>in warmth and in grace,
>and learns that abundance
>was never a race.

3.5 Healing My Warrior Protector

> She rose from the ashes
> with fire in her chest,
> a sword made of silence,
> a shield built from stress.
>
> She marched without resting,
> with grit in her grace,
> fighting for safety
> in every lost place.
>
> But now she's invited
> to soften her stance,
> to lay down the armor
> and give peace a chance.

Most children exposed to parental abuse or neglect grow up fearing to voice their needs, concerns, and disappointments, often to avoid further harm. This was the case for my inner child. When the seeds of doubt began to crack the idealized image she held of her parents, my *warrior protective part* came to life. Her mission was to speak up, protect my inner child by giving voice to her pain. This part is always alert, even if not always visible. She is fearless and ready to defend my inner child in any way necessary.

In her childhood home, voices were either loud and overbearing or silent and submissive. My inner child chose silence, absorbing accusations and enduring toxic criticism without protest. Yet deep within, she longed to fight back, to defend herself from those who ignored or belittled her. Though, my warrior part's voice was hesitant at first. For many years, she feared making my inner child feel guilty for speaking up and was unsure how to be effective. Her early expressions reflected victimhood and a desire to awaken compassion from her parents. But those early efforts were met with invalidation, blame, and more conditions. Sometimes she tried brief, witty remarks instead, sarcasm, subtle mirrors to help others see their behaviour. Her sister, in particular, began to recognize these sharp observations. Still, this warrior part wasn't always equipped to respond appropriately to every situation. Her wisdom and strength took time to grow.

As she began to realize that her family wasn't listening, her approach shifted. She became more forceful. At times, when being under attack, she raised her voice, named the harm, and stood her ground when she noticed that the overgiving part didn't feel appreciated. Instead of remorse or repair, she was met with defensiveness and retaliation. They weaponized her honesty, projecting their insecurities and using manipulation to regain control through guilt, fear, and shame.

One significant moment came when she confronted my father about a call I received in high school, asking whether he had cheated on my mother. His immediate deflection, accusing *her* of cheating, confirmed more than his infidelity. It showed his complete inability to own his actions. In that moment, my warrior part chose silence. At his old age, if he still felt the need to tarnish a woman who could no longer defend herself, no argument could bring clarity. She saw no point in playing his blame game.

From experiences like these, my warrior part learned a vital truth: you cannot argue someone into empathy and honesty. It's a waste of energy to try to change self-absorbed people who are not willing to change and, unfortunately, most of them don't. The more she faced these situations, the more she realized that walking away was the most effective way to communicate with self-absorbed people. Walking away became her most effective defence; silence not as weakness, but as strength. She learned that silence could be a powerful form of protest, a way to say *I see you, but I choose peace.* She realized that true strength wasn't in proving her wrong, but in recognizing that she didn't need anyone's approval to feel secure in her truth. Walking away from those arguments wasn't a defeat; it was a quiet victory, one that honoured my time, energy, and emotional boundaries.

Undoing reactivity hasn't been easy. Even though she hasn't always been reactive. There have been many times when the urge to *tell her truth* felt overwhelming. But she learned that in many cases, restraint held more power. She now takes time to evaluate the situation, the person, and the history, especially how they responded to constructive feedback in the past. She understands that not every person or moment deserves the same response.

Since the collective decided to remove toxic people from my inner child's life, there have been times when some of them tried to return. My warrior part takes on the responsibility of discerning their intentions. Genuine remorse is shown through meaningful apologies, consistent actions, and respect for boundaries, not vague texts, half-hearted questions, or invitations that ignore the past. She's learned that when people break boundaries and pretend nothing happened, it's a red flag, not a sign of love or change. If a connection ended for a valid reason and the damage remained unaddressed, she feels no obligation to re-engage. Sometimes, the best response is *no response at all.*

One of her greatest lessons has been this: *How a person responds to "no" reveals the truth about their intentions.* Self-absorbed people don't take "no" lightly. They may stalk, harass, manipulate, write bad reviews about your business hoping to ruin your reputation and financial stability, or choose even more harmful actions. To them, every interaction is a power struggle. If they once held power, they want it back, and any resistance feels like defiance. The consistency of the *no-contact rule* is essential. This rule is not about revenge, it's about protecting the peace and dignity my inner child has earned.

She no longer believes it's her job to make herself understood by those who refuse to listen. She doesn't need to shout, plead, or argue. Silence now speaks volumes. It communicates her worth. And she knows consistency is key, because any inconsistency can be twisted by the manipulative parts of others.

Despite this growth, the early stages of healing brought anger. My warrior part was furious with herself. *"I knew what they were doing... They didn't fool me!"* She felt she had failed to protect the inner child. Her voice was valid, her instincts were right, but other parts didn't listen. Nothing could undo those past decisions. The only option left was to communicate better going forward.

She also experienced resentment toward those who hurt her inner child. Her anger stirred a longing for justice, not revenge, but transformation. She hoped those people would experience something that would wake them up, encourage them to reflect, and bring healing to their own inner child. However, she cannot deny that she wanted them to *acknowledge* the pain they had caused to her inner child.

My Self embraced these emotions, knowing they were real and worthy of acknowledgment. But over time, my warrior part recognized that clinging to anger and blame only harmed her. It added stress to an already heavy burden. Through spiritual reflection and the Self's guidance, she came to understand that *justice is always served*, even if it's not visible right away. No wrongdoing is overlooked.

This memoir is part of that justice. She wants to share this story with others who are vulnerable to the same kind of abuse to empower them to find their voice, boundaries, and peace.

>She fought so long
>no one saw her ache
>protecting the child
>with every move she'd make.
>
>Now she stands softer,
>not weaker, but wise
>a warrior who's learning
>to walk away and rest.

3.6 Healing My Overgiving Protector

> She gave too much,
> too fast, too soon,
> her hands were full
> beneath the moon.
>
> A child inside
> still hoped they'd see
> that giving love
> would set her free.

Of course, there's a part of me who used to overgive. Her role was to protect and love my inner child. This part is as old as the inner child herself, a personality trait she was born with. In her eyes, love meant caring for others. She was groomed by her parents to be humble, compliant, reliable, and never complain. Her intention was always to offer unconditional love and build nice connections with others that would soothe her inner child. To some extent, I believe this part's belief system was shaped by her mother's stories related to her childhood and the ones read by my inner child, stories where unselfish, loving characters healed others through their kindness. In those stories, love always triumphed.

Vulnerability was never something she avoided. On the contrary, she embraced it, believing it fostered a deep emotional connection. Throughout life, she expressed love through kind words, hugs, kisses, baking, cooking, and sacrificing her own needs. This protector truly believed that the kindness she would give to others would return to her inner child. As a child, she saved her lunch money for weeks to buy her mother's favourite perfume for her birthday, because loving and protecting those close to her inner child came naturally.

Despite her gentleness and altruism, this part has always played a dominant role among my other protectors, especially when abandonment pain was triggered. She not only wanted to prevent that pain from resurfacing but also carefully evaluated her actions to shield the inner child. Her desire to build a loving home and family for her inner child influenced many decisions. And in doing so, she often silenced the other protective parts, unable to see how her dominance was denying the inner child's real needs, and exposing her to people who took advantage of her generosity.

It was only after realizing that her altruism had become an expectation, that her love was not reciprocated but taken for granted, that she began to understand the consequences of her choices. Change didn't happen all at once. Her healing has been a slow, gradual process that hasn't ended. It involved learning to set boundaries with the people she loved the most. Though it felt too overwhelming to do it with everyone at once.

It took years to see how even her blood related family had exploited her kindness. And once she recognized this, she still didn't understand well the nature of their struggles, and the guilt ingrained by her parents weighed heavily on her. Before moving to Canada, she confided in a priest, seeking advice as guilt consumed her. To her surprise, he supported her decision, urging her to allow her inner child to live her own life. That moment became a turning point. Though painful, she pushed through the guilt and accepted that her parents were focused solely on themselves. Her family expected her to fulfill the role of a *"good child"*, dictating how that role should be carried.

Then, it wasn't entirely clear that she was being used by other people as well. Abuse by self-centred individuals often goes unnoticed, it's subtle, a cycle of love and cruelty that creates confusion and false hope. She feared causing others the same pain her inner child endured by not being accepted or seen. Gradually, they held her accountable for their well-being and she chose silence over the well-being of her own inner child. Eventually, she felt drained. Giving love only to be met with manipulation and disdain left her empty. The pain of her inner child became unbearable, built up over the years. That pain became a wake-up call for this healing process for her and many other protective parts. She could no longer live like this. Her inner child deserved more. She deserved peace, love, and freedom.

Self-blame came in waves once healing began. *"How did this happen? How could they hurt my inner child so much?"* she asked. She had every reason to question things, after all, she continued loving them, trusting their empty promises. But those questions brought no healing. To truly grow, she had to ask new ones: "*What can I do to protect my inner child now?*", "*What lessons have I learned from these experiences?*"

Healing came through recognizing her inner child's worth and understanding that others are responsible for their own healing. She saw that suppressing guilt didn't make it go away. It was a survival strategy. Now, instead of feeling guilty for prioritizing her inner child, she makes choices that nurture her well-being. She allowed other protective parts to have a voice.

When speaking to her family, she started using "*I*" on behalf of her inner child. "I *deserve to breathe for myself.*" "*I am worthy of love.*" She didn't abandon her family; they abandoned themselves and her inner child as well. She redefined family as those who love with open hearts, not necessarily those connected by blood.

The recent changes she made caused ripples, helping her see that she had crafted an illusion for her inner child, a hopeful belief that others would see and value her with the same depth and tenderness she offered them. But they didn't. When she stopped giving, the truth began to reveal itself. The act of withdrawing revealed the imbalance that was always there, masked by her effort to maintain connection. It became clear how they viewed her, not as a whole person with needs of her own, but as someone whose role was to give, accommodate, fill gaps they never intended to address themselves. Some demanded the same care, pushed against her boundaries, or protested her silence. Others didn't even notice her absence until later and claimed to feel confused by this change in her behavior. Some people backed away, unable to accept her growth. Others tried to manipulate her into returning to her old ways, using especially emotional blackmail. Not one reflected on their actions, offered a heartfelt apology, or showed genuine concern for the well-being of her inner child.

In this new space, her overgiving part no longer takes responsibility for these people's reactions. Their energy no longer matches hers. She's learned that love includes boundaries, that saying "no" can be an act of love.

Reflecting on her past hasn't been easy. She sees how much she gave to people who did not value her. She offered them years of love and dedication, only to be met with silence, disrespect, and emotional neglect. Her mother cursed her instead of soothing her. Her father never reached out to her, though she called him regularly. Still, her inner child held onto them with love, even after seeing their true selves.

From this pain came clarity: she will now choose carefully who enters her life. Her decisions aren't based on black-and-white thinking, but on the undeniable truth of repeated harm. She understands that no one is perfect; we all lose our temper and make mistakes. But those who truly care take responsibility, apologize, and try to grow. The self-absorbed people don't.

She intends to evaluate other people's actions before giving second chances. She no longer seeks to prove her inner child's worth or gain external validation. What others think of this journey doesn't matter; they didn't live it. She understands that everyone is responsible for their own healing. While she offers compassion, it's reserved for the wounded inner child in others, not for the parts that knowingly cause harm.

This part of me has been practicing forgiveness, not just for others, but for herself. Forgiveness is a gift of freedom and peace. In the past, she equated forgiveness with forgetting and minimizing harm. Now she knows that by ignoring harmful behaviour, she abandoned her inner child. True forgiveness honours the pain and refuses to let it dictate the future. She recognizes how the people she loved had used her love as a weapon. She no longer allows that.

Writing this memoir helped her understand herself more deeply - why she made certain decisions, some painful, others profound. Not everything she did was a mistake. She offered genuine love to others, some of whom may have, because of her, gained at least a fleeting understanding of what true love is. At the time, loving others felt effortless. For a long time, she believed it was effortless for everyone.

Now, she is learning to forgive at her own pace. She honours every emotion: sadness, anger, grief, as part of her journey. Forgiveness doesn't mean forgetting. It means remembering clearly, so the same harm is never allowed again.

Today, her overgiving part is committed to protecting her inner child's dreams. Love exists within her.

She still gives,
but not to lose
her worth no longer
others choose.

Now rooted deep
in sacred ground,
she shares from wholeness,
not to be found.

3.7 Healing My Inner Critics

They wake when shadows stretch too long,
Whispers riding the edges of my thoughts.
"You're not enough," they chant, relentless,
Echoes of a world that demanded perfection.

They measure each step, each word, each breath,
Counting mistakes that never were meant to exist.
Yet beneath the sharpened edges, a trembling heart
Fearful, tender, trying to shield the small child inside.

They push, they prod, they build invisible walls,
A fortress of vigilance around a fragile self.
And though I stumble under their weight,
I feel the love hidden in their discipline.

For in their harshness lies a hope:
That I might escape the sting they once knew,
That I might walk, unshaken,
Through a world that once punished me for being.

All my critical protective parts emerged early in life as a result of my inner child absorbing the projections of her family members' insecurities. At night, when the voices of ridicule echoed in her mind, calling her "*stupid*," mocking her words, and questioning her worth, these parts came alive. They began second-guessing her thoughts and actions, urging her to strive for better in the future, hoping to shield her from further rejection or criticism. Whenever my inner child didn't know whether her decisions would satisfy her mother's desires, my inner critics would replay past conversations, trying to decipher what she had done "wrong" and how she could avoid triggering anger. They internalized the meanings my inner child gave to her experiences and built strategies to help her survive, always scanning for ways to stay safe.

Over time, these critical parts became relentless taskmasters, driving my inner child to meet impossibly high standards. They whispered doubts disguised as warnings - *"You're not good enough," "You must try harder," "Don't make mistakes"* - fueling a cycle of self-judgment and striving. Yet, beneath their harshness lay a protective impulse: they believed that by pushing harder, they could prevent the pain of rejection and abandonment that had shaped the experiences of their inner child.

Though these parts often felt like enemies, they were rooted in fear and care. They carried the heavy burden of my family's unspoken rules - rules about perfection, obedience, and invisibility. My inner critics learned to be alert, ready to adapt and survive in an environment where mistakes were punished and love was conditional. Without them, my inner child might have felt even more vulnerable and alone.

As healing was initiated, my Self invited them into dialogue and reminded them that their role could evolve - that protection didn't require punishment, and love didn't have to be earned.

3.7.1 The Obedient Protector

She learned to bow before the storm,
to keep the peace, to change her form.
A whispered "sorry" held the weight
of years spent trying to navigate
the moods of those who called it "love,"
yet raged and ruled from far above.

But now she speaks, not to appease,
her voice a wind that dares to breathe.

One critical protective part became obsessed with evaluating how much "*love*" and "*respect*" her inner child had shown to her parents and sister, words heavily emphasized in their household. From the beginning, this part learned to adapt by reading others' needs and avoiding conflict, because my inner child feared confrontation. My inner child often walked on eggshells to avoid unpredictable outbursts that created fear. My obedient part wanted to smooth the path and protect her from pain. She has always been able to sense her other people's emotional distress and sought to soothe it with love and obedience. She learned to navigate difficult situations by mastering the art of obedience: saying "*sorry*," staying silent, following imposed rules, appeasing demands, and taking the blame without protest when others wanted to be always "*right*.". She learned to navigate life among individuals with self-absorption traits by anticipating dissatisfaction and avoiding it at all costs.

This obedient part was never alone in her work. She moved in tandem with your overgiving part, both of them fluent in the unspoken rule: *If I give enough, stay quiet enough, please well enough - maybe I'll be safe. Maybe I'll be loved.* Their strategies were aligned, refined over years of walking on emotional eggshells. One smoothed the surface with silence; the other with sacrifice. But while their methods differed in flavor, their purpose was the same: protect the inner child from rejection, chaos, and pain. Still, the system was never static.

Decades ago, when the warrior part began to rise, slowly, defiantly, something shifted. The warrior didn't ask for permission to exist and didn't apologize for speaking the truth. And the obedient part watched with awe. Alongside her, the highly functioning part emerged too, not to perform or perfect, but to *stabilize*. She began building a life with structure and strength.This part didn't rely on obedience or overgiving, but on competence, consistency, and vision. For the obedient part, this was the beginning of transformation. No longer isolated in her survival strategy, she began to feel the stirrings of trust in other protectors, in strength, in a system that no longer required her to bow to stay safe.

Though she had walked beside the overgiving part for many years, she was the first to set herself free. Freedom didn't arrive all at once, it came in small acts of defiance against the roles she had once depended on. It showed up in moments where she chose to pause instead of please, to stay instead of shrink, to speak instead of apologize. At first, it felt unnatural, even wrong. Her nervous system flinched at the absence of control, of preemptive peacekeeping. But with each choice, she loosened the grip of old beliefs: that love must be earned, that safety comes through silence, that survival depends on surrendering one's truth.

This protector began to sense that her worth had never been tied to obedience. That her inner child didn't need to perform goodness to deserve care. And with that realization, the obedient part softened. She no longer had to brace for rejection or anticipate every emotional shift in the room. She didn't vanish; she transformed. From a servant of fear to a guardian of boundaries. From a peacekeeper in chaos to an advocate for self-respect and gender equality.

And perhaps most beautifully, she became a bridge. One who could extend compassion to the overgiving part still learning to assess and choose her responsibilities, how to let go, and who she wanted to become. Knowing what it felt like to serve without rest, to love without limits, she didn't judge her, but offered her something different: a whisper that they could change their old alliance into something new based on mutual reflection, shared accountability, and a shared willingness to grow. Together, they began offering insight to other parts still caught in outdated roles.

This part is no longer just the obedient one. She's the harmonizer. Not because she keeps the peace at any cost, but because now, she knows the difference between forced peace and true harmony.

She swallowed words to keep things calm,
wrapped tension tight inside her palm.
She bowed to blame, absorbed the heat,
called silence, love and guilt, her seat.

But now she whispers, firm and free:
"I owe no penance just to be."

3.7.2 The Negotiator Protector

> She stitched her heart with silken thread,
> a tapestry of hope and dread.
> "If I give enough," she softly cried,
> "maybe love won't run and hide."
>
> She bartered truth to keep the peace,
> made self-worth small so pain would cease.
> She taught the child to dim her light,
> to trade her voice for being liked.
>
> But quiet bargains cost too much -
> a hunger grows in absence's clutch.
> And love, she learned, must not be bought -
> nor should it leave us overwrought.

She was born in the silence that followed abandonment. When the voices that once called me "daughter" faded, when love turned conditional or disappeared altogether, this part stepped forward. Not with loud resistance, but with quiet resolve. She couldn't undo what had been done, couldn't mend the fracture that left my inner child alone and aching. But she could *do something*. And so, she took on the impossible task of protecting a wounded heart in a world that had already proven its unreliability.

Her method was subtle but relentless: lower expectations, raise tolerance. She was a master of reframing, of ignoring people's hurtful actions and focusing on someone's potential instead, concealing a deeper, more painful belief: that my inner child was unlovable.

Like many children who experience parental rejection, she internalized the idea that she might never find someone who would truly love her. When her parents left, she didn't assume they were flawed; instead, she assumed *she* was. This protective part tried to shield her by lowering expectations of others. When red flags appeared in her relationships, she focused on the good aspects, making excuses for the rest. Over time, the discomfort in these connections became familiar. She began negotiating what was tolerable, adjusting to pain as if it were normal. In doing so, she wasn't helping my inner child see her value; she was compromising it.

But she didn't do this to harm her. Like all protective parts, she longed for my inner child to experience real love. But this strategy came with a heavy cost. She simply fell into the trap of negotiating self-worth in exchange for closeness. Each time she negotiated away our needs, each time she softened a red flag or buried a boundary, she carved a deeper distance between us and our own worth. My inner child, already wounded, began to believe she had to *earn* what should have been freely given. That she had to inspire love, not simply receive it.

Once the healing journey began, everything changed. Sacrificing sovereignty was no longer acceptable. When forced to choose between solitude and unhealthy connections, this part chose to stand with the other protective parts, committing to peace over dysfunction. She recognized my inner child's right to be respected and unconditionally loved. This part also came to understand how important it is to avoid people who evoke the same feelings that her family's mistreatment once triggered. Familiarity doesn't always mean safety. Now, this part safeguards space for relationships that are nourishing, reciprocal, and emotionally safe.

My inner child longs for connection, people to laugh with in joy, cry with in pain, and share life's precious moments. We are meant to lean on others, to be seen, supported, understood, and not live in isolation. Though, my inner child should never again have to *earn* love by fixing others, motivating them, boosting the self-esteem of their inner child, or becoming the target of their projections. She deserves relationships with people who are emotionally consistent, who can see beyond their own needs, and who respect differences without turning them into battles. She deserves people who are capable of giving as much as they receive.

> Now she stands where pain once led,
> a crown of knowing on her head.
> No longer bending, soft, or blind
> she guards the worth we've come to find.
>
> She sees the signs, she knows the tone,
> the way that chaos feels like home.

And when old patterns call us near,
she speaks with strength, not shame or fear.

"This child," she says, "is not a cure.
She's not a balm for hearts unsure.
She won't be shaped by someone's lack
she's whole, and I won't send her back."

3.7.3 The Underminer Protector

> She kept me small to keep me safe,
> a quiet ghost who knew her place.
> She whispered doubt to block the pain,
> afraid that truth would bring disdain.
>
> But now she speaks with steady grace,
> a voice that knows it has a place.

Another part, the underminer, emerged in early childhood during moments of conflict. When others projected feelings of inferiority onto my inner child, this part adapted by internalizing those messages. She began undermining the child's confidence, suppressing her voice to prevent rejection, and attempting to keep her small to avoid scrutiny. Her voice carried anxiety, especially while living with her parents. Even rehearsing her words couldn't quiet the fear of being misunderstood.

Her healing began when challenged by my highly functioning part, a determined force who continually urged growth. At first, the underminer resisted, afraid of risk. But over time, witnessing the determination of the high-functioning part to create a better life, she began to help. She learned her role could evolve. By embracing vulnerability, she allowed her inner child to express herself, even imperfectly. That act alone was liberating.

Over the decades, trust blossomed between these two parts. The underminer developed confidence, and her voice grew strong, capable of expressing needs, setting boundaries, and even offering constructive feedback. Her transformation brought the collective closer to authenticity and autonomy. Her role shifted from suppression to empowerment.

Once she trembled at the sound
of truth too loud, of thoughts unbound.
But courage grew, not loud, but deep -
a seed that cracked the shell of "keep."

Now she stands, no longer less
a voice reborn in bold express.

3.7.4 The Destroyer of Ancestral Trauma Protector

> She saw the thread that tied the past,
> each silent vow, each shadow cast.
> She didn't flinch or turn away
> she rose to burn the rot away.
>
> Not out of hate, but love so wide:
> *This ends with me,* she said, and cried.

Another vital protective part emerged when my inner child began rejecting her family's dysfunctional behaviours. This part took on the role of the vigilant examiner, constantly scanning for signs that any internalized behaviours might mirror those of her family. She carried within her the hunger for love untainted by manipulation, for relationships grounded in mutual respect rather than control. Unlike the other protectors, who learned to survive by conforming to the family's rules, she longed to break free of them. She whispered to the inner child that life could be different, that values like authenticity, tenderness, and truth could replace shame, fear, and silence.

This protector challenged the inherited beliefs of obedience, self-sacrifice, and invisibility. She questioned why love had to be conditional, why individuality had to be punished, and why loyalty to the family required betraying oneself. Though she often appeared destructive, dismantling what seemed stable, her destruction carried purpose. She sought to clear the ground where something new could grow: relationships not defined by hierarchy, but by love; identities not molded by fear, but by freedom.

Her fire was the refusal to accept that the family's way was the only way. She carried the dream of another path, one her inner child longed for but could not yet walk alone. She was driven by a deep desire to prevent harm, ensure accountability, and break the cycle of inherited trauma. She is the one who promised to herself that she would never give up on her child. Therefore, this part acted as a vigilant observer, carefully examining interpersonal dynamics and parenting patterns within the system. She questioned motives, uncovered hidden patterns, and held a clear vision for breaking harmful cycles.

From an early age, she dreamed of becoming a teacher, creating an internal code for how she would speak to every child, ensuring her words would never inflict psychological harm. Her deepest desire was always to empower children and young people. Guided by this mission, she influenced my other protective parts to remain attentive to a child's emotions, making certain that no one ever felt overlooked, abandoned, or unworthy.

At times, her voice was quite strong and initially was met with resistance, as some parts felt uncomfortable being evaluated so critically. Though at first she struggled to connect with all parts, her persistence led to honest internal dialogues. Through these conversations, the collective recognized that, while some of their behaviours were maladaptive, the core intentions of the parts had always been to protect.

Eventually, the system accepted this part as a crucial ally. Her feedback became constructive, offering insights that helped refine each part's protective strategy to better align with the Self. Her unwavering commitment to integrity and transformation became a guiding light in the healing process.

Her goal has never been to blame, but to find the truth. By helping the collective understand the pain of the past and dismantle inherited patterns, she ensured the system wouldn't unconsciously repeat what it was once subjected to. Her role has been vital in the collective's evolution toward clarity, accountability, and inner peace.

> She once stayed small to not offend,
> her silence bent, afraid to bend.
> Each thought rehearsed, each word a test,
> shrinking, she believed she'd rest.
>
> But healing called her to the light -
> to rise, to name, to claim her right.
> Now doubt gives way to something new:
> a self who knows her worth is true.

3.8 **Meeting my Self**

Underneath our Sun, we all are walking the Earth making steps through our Life...

Some of us are running, desperately searching for majesty,

Some are taking one step at a time,

Smelling flowers, grass and looking into people's eyes...

Underneath our Clouds, we are all searching for the little home of Happiness...

A place where people hug, heal and lean on each other,

where People have the Sun Dance...

A place where being is about connection,

not about possessions,

where snakes, mountains and people are all interconnected...

Underneath our Surface, we need to be Free...

Some of us are looking for freedom to conquer, no matter what,

Some others are just trying to feel free with

themselves in their touching songs,

in their consciousness,

In exploring their spirituality...

Underneath our Will Power, there is Desire ....

to connect with ourselves... sometimes even in
our last moments of our lives,

to face our fears and to connect in every step we take
through our Life....

Underneath Everything, there is You...

It is You in the act of showing sympathy for all beings,

of staying silent to listen to what others may say,

of respecting their LIVES,

of learning not to chase other people's thoughts,

But connect with their way of being, talking and living...

Stop...

Surrender...

Allow yourself to Love...

External pressures can cloud our judgment, pulling us away from our true essence. Yet the truth of who we are has always lived within us. When we reconnect with it, the experience is both profound and invigorating. This inner truth becomes a compass, guiding us through internal storms, clearing away energetic blocks, and helping us release what no longer serves our inner child. Once that connection is made, the path forward becomes unmistakable and almost impossible to abandon. It transforms the way we see life. It brings us back to ourselves.

My Self is wise, values compassion, peace, kindness, honesty, life, creativity, accountability, clarity, stability, authenticity, empowerment, and creativity. She values justice, but not through her hands.

To access my Self, I practice metacognition, the skill of observing one's thoughts, and mindfulness. At first, I ground myself through mindfulness, which offers a safe space to find calmness amidst inner chaos. Within that calm, the Self emerges, steady and non-reactive, simply observing the waves of thoughts and emotions without judgment. The emotions and thoughts that surface in this space belong to protective parts that are asking to be seen. With compassion, my Self invites these parts into dialogue. Gently, it asks questions: What is your role? What pain gave birth to you? What have you been trying to protect? With patience and curiosity, the Self listened-not to fix or silence them, but to understand.

These reflective moments have helped identify not only the purpose of each part but also the stories they carried - stories born from fear, loneliness, or unmet needs. The Self didn't dismiss them; instead, it helped these parts evaluate whether their protective strategies still served the well-being of the inner child. Often, resolving their struggles meant inviting other parts into collaboration, showing them that healing didn't need to be a solo mission, but a shared journey led by trust and understanding.

My Self values authenticity, not as a performance or ideal, but as a way of being that honours truth, integrity, and inner alignment. Authenticity, to her, is fully embraced when the inner child and her protective parts refuse to carry the projections others place on them. It is felt when they no longer shrink to fit into environments shaped by other people's protective parts, or contort themselves just to feel accepted.

The power of authenticity is cultivated through self-awareness, by inviting each protective part to reflect on the coping strategies they developed in the past, and gently guiding them to evaluate whether those strategies still serve the inner child's growth and wellbeing. The Self doesn't force change; but invites for collaboration. The Self honours their history and encourages evolution. As each part has come into alignment with the values of the Self, such as integrity, compassion, courage, and freedom, authenticity becomes not only possible but inevitable. It becomes the natural expression of a system that is not driven by fear or shame, but guided by clarity, love, and trust.

The journey of guiding my inner child and her protective parts is, in itself, the truest reward of this lifetime. This path brings the justice they have longed for, not through external validation or revenge, but through deep transformation and self-leadership. Although the journey has felt heavy at times, it holds profound meaning because every step forward is a step toward reclaiming her worth. There is immense power in watching each protective part grow in self-awareness, learning to attune to the subtle cues the Self sends, recognizing whether their actions align or stray from the values of the Self. This process builds trust. It builds inner unity. And with each layer of understanding, the potential for deeper healing and expansion reveals itself.

Justice is no longer something to be found outside. It emerges from within, from the growing resilience of this internal collective. Every painful experience becomes a lesson that sharpens their ability to decode others' behaviours with more clarity and discernment. This insight offers protection, not from a place of fear, but from love, the kind that finally knows how to guard what was once left unprotected.

My Self is deeply proud of her collective, proud of their unwavering commitment to seek clarity about their past beliefs and desires, speak their truth, and share their unique perspective with the world. She sees within them a vast potential for continued transformation.

My inner child's protective parts resisted change at first. Some clung to control or retreated into familiar worlds built to avoid the pain of reality. But over time, they surrendered. They began to honour their imperfections. They allowed space for reflection and owned the deep desire to live differently. In doing so, they chose a path aligned not just with survival, but with healing and growth. A path that resonates with their evolving goals, values, and capacity to care for the child they once couldn't protect very well.

While sitting in stillness and trust, my protective parts and inner child allowed what needed to arise to be seen. My Self, quietly present, acknowledged their courage and resilience, their efforts to face the pain and navigate the challenges they once believed they had to carry alone. Their wounds were met with kindness, and in return, they received the gentle wisdom that only compassion can bring. One by one, they've been learning to align with the values of my Self, allowing vulnerability, honouring their positive intentions, embracing their imperfections, and cultivating deeper self-awareness. Together, they've committed to improving their communication, building trust, and supporting each other more intentionally in the future. In their unity, my Self sees the quiet power of transformation, not as a destination, but as a deepening journey home.

By listening to the quiet voice of my Self, they learned to communicate with honesty and intention. United by a common purpose, they chose to support my inner child in reclaiming her power, not through resistance, but through clarity, compassion, and truth. They came to understand that this was their chance to protect her, not just from the past, but from future wounds that might arise. Guided gently by my Self, they began working together to create something strong and enduring: a shield. That shield is self-love. And when others try to penetrate this shield, as there are always people who push boundaries and seek only to receive, they now recognize the signs more quickly. They no longer act impulsively or betray their own needs. They pause, reflect, and protect. Because they know the cost of abandoning the inner child. And they choose, again and again, to protect her instead.

Through the guidance of my Self, my protective parts learned to shed past behaviours and treat themselves with kindness and gentleness. Practices like self-care, meditation, Reiki, positive affirmations, and staying connected to their Self helped bring peace within and among them.

This deepened understanding of my inner world has led to more cohesive choices, greater compassion, and lasting harmony. While life hasn't paused during this healing, the Universe has tested the strength they've built. Even when challenged, my parts no longer reacted impulsively or in isolation. Now, they understand one another's triggers. The guilt and shame they once carried began to dissolve as they recognized their own *"super traits"*, qualities like agreeableness and conscientiousness, common among survivors of self-absorbed people. In time, these emotions faded completely.

My Self truly believes in the power of love. Unconditional love. Love is our direct link to the Universe. Self-love brings balance and peace. I am working on bringing balance and peace into my life every day. Some days it feels effortless, as if the Universe is holding my hand and guiding me toward grace. On other days, grief is very much present, whispering reminders of the past and the losses I have carried. Yet even then, I choose to love myself in the midst of the ache. I offer tenderness to the parts of me still mourning, and I extend love outward to others, because love does not disappear when pain arrives. If anything, it deepens, becoming richer and more compassionate, like light filtering through rain.

The more my parts have begun to trust the guidance of my Self, the more they have awakened. This awakening has been a gradual, unfolding process. One of my protective parts, ever skeptical, kept questioning these experiences. Through this connection, my Self found the exact resources that could soothe the wounds of my inner child and bring clarity to my protective parts. This is how they've found resources that changed everything - Internal Family Systems Therapy, Brainspotting - quantum music, insights about cognitive dissonance, and abuse from self-absorbed people. None of this healing would have been possible in the same way without the guidance of the Universe. These resources became the language through which my Self could reach my parts, and together, we began to come home to ourselves.

My inner child and her protectors remembered many other events from her life that once felt unexplainable: strange coincidences, quiet nudges, intuitive decisions, things that didn't make sense at the time. But they began to take shape and reveal their meaning as my inner child and protective parts moved closer to my Self.

Then, one day, my inner child found something remarkable, a note I had written to my inner child more than thirty years ago. She was too young to recognize my voice at the time.

"It would be too trivial to ask God to give you what you lost, but I ask Him to give you strength in the future to get through the most difficult moments of your life."

At the time, my inner child didn't fully understand what those words meant, only that they brought comfort, like a whisper from something deep within her. Now she hears the voice of her Self - timeless and ever-present, reaching across decades to plant a seed of resilience. That single sentence held the essence of everything she needed to remember: that she couldn't rewrite the past, but she could carry strength into the future. That note has become a symbol of the deep, unwavering guidance that has always been within her, the first evidence that her Self never left her, even when the world felt far too heavy to carry.

When she was little, my inner child shared a close and beautiful bond with her Self, a quiet connection that revealed itself in subtle, magical ways. On several occasions, her Self would send her intuitive whispers and communicate with her through vivid dreams. In a few pivotal moments, when she stood at life's crossroads, my Self gently whispered to her, urging her to consider a different path, one that promised more depth, more meaning, and more authentic connections. These nudges weren't vague; they carried a clear sense of direction. My Self even revealed glimpses of the outcome that would follow the path that felt most tempting to her heart.

Despite feeling protected through many difficult times, as if a powerful force was always watching over her, my inner child didn't yet recognize this voice as the wisdom of her Self. She didn't know that it was her inner compass gently trying to steer her toward wholeness. Instead, she chose to follow the voice of her heart, a heart full of longing, hope, and the deep desire to be loved. Only recently did my inner child finally come to recognize that quiet, unwavering voice, the one that had always been there, whispering truths and offering clarity. It was the voice of her Self. Now, my inner child wonders if our Self holds a deeper wisdom than we are currently able to access. Maybe, through higher levels of consciousness, we can tap into the full knowledge that the Self carries.

But through these moments, my inner child and her protectors began to understand just how powerful thoughts truly are. They shape the reality we live in. If we believe we are not lovable, not enough, we unconsciously make decisions that affirm those beliefs. We attract people in our life that reflect those doubts back to us. Even when we recognize red flags, we may still feel unable to leave, as these beliefs cloud our connection to the Self and to the wisdom of the Universe.

Empathy, for instance, can create connection and intimacy when balanced. But too much empathy, especially when misdirected, can lead to burnout, people-pleasing, and relationships with those who demand constant attention to fill their inner voids. When we take on others' struggles and allow their pain to become our own, we amplify negative thoughts within ourselves - thoughts that become self-fulfilling, trapping us in a reality that feels harder and harder to escape. When we believe those thoughts, they shape our choices. They build a life around fear. That's not mysticism, it's a fact.

On the other hand, when our thoughts are positive, our inner child and protective parts feel safe, grounded, and free to co-create with the Universe. In those moments, there is no resistance. Instead, there is flow. When my inner child and her protective parts matched the frequency of my Self, they found a profound sense of peace, joy, and safety. In this state of harmony, they no longer felt the need to chase healing or fix the past. They were simply able to be fully present, without pressure or fear.

There were no expectations imposed from within or outside. My inner child no longer felt like she had to perform, prove herself, or meet invisible standards to be loved or accepted. And in that space of clarity, she released the resentment she once held toward those who had hurt her. That pain no longer defined her story. Yet, even without forgetting, she didn't feel the need to stop loving them either. This is the peace that comes when we live in alignment with our Self, when we remember who we truly are, beyond the protective layers we've built to survive. It's not detachment or denial, it's liberation. It's the freedom to love without losing ourselves.

My Self values compassion and practices forgiveness, not as an invitation for others to reenter and repeat harm, but as a release from the burden of holding onto resentment. As long as those who once hurt her inner child do not attempt to return and cause further pain, my Self wishes them well on their own journey.

She hopes they one day find their way back to their own Self, and that they rediscover the beauty and innocence of their own inner child, the part of them that also deserves love, protection, and tenderness. That part didn't deserve the suffering it endured. And while it may have learned to protect itself in ways that hurt others, it too, longs for peace.

Their Self, when they are ready to listen, can guide them to break free from the illusions they've constructed. Illusions of power, control, or admiration that ultimately leave them empty. My Self knows that true peace cannot be built by clinging to other people's energy, love, or resources. That form of survival may provide temporary comfort, but it will never be enough. It only reflects the deeper illusion: the illusion that they are truly loved.

To find real joy, they must stop trying to mirror others and instead turn inward. Only by stepping out of survival mode and into self-awareness can they discover the love they've been seeking all along, the love of their own Self.

> I am the stillness in the storm,
> the gentle light, the quiet form.
> Not born of fear, nor shaped by pain,
> but rising soft like morning rain.
>
> I hold the parts, both fierce and shy,
> and whisper truths that never die.
> In me, they rest - no need to strive,
> for I am love, and I'm alive.

Part II – Understanding Self-Absorption Through IFS lens

Chapter 4

The internal landscape of self-absorbed people seen through the lens of IFS therapy

In this chapter, I sought to highlight the shared experiences, thoughts, emotions, psychological responses, and behaviors often present in people with self-absorbed tendencies. Through patterns I've observed both personally and professionally, I have attempted to decode the struggles of the wounded inner child within these individuals, along with the protective parts that arose to shield them in response to unmet needs. These patterns should not be interpreted as depictions of any specific individual.

What emerged was a kind of psychological kaleidoscope, a mosaic of protective parts, each with distinct roles, yet deeply interconnected. These parts reveal complex internal dynamics, not only within the individuals themselves but also in how they relate to others. This understanding has been invaluable to my healing. Recognizing these patterns has empowered me to approach future encounters with greater awareness and emotional clarity. I hope this information will help you too.

My intention here is not to shame these individuals. I recognize that their protective parts were activated to safeguard a wounded inner child. Though I've suffered from their actions, I hold compassion for that inner child. I do not wish to harm them. Instead, I see those protective parts for what they are: survival strategies that formed in the absence of love, safety, and emotional attunement who are harming others and have no remorse for doing so. I still hold hope that, if they choose to embrace gentleness, curiosity, vulnerability, self-compassion, and authentic love, healing is possible for them too.

While this memoir is written primarily for those who have suffered from the behaviours of self-absorbed individuals, it's important to acknowledge that many of these self-absorbed individuals carry wounds remarkably similar to mine, particularly the deep pain of parental abandonment. The difference is that many of their protective parts remain deeply entrenched in denial, purposely harm others, see themselves as superior to others and seem to be blind to the harm they cause, not only to others but also to their inner child.

Perhaps, in sharing my perspective and understanding of their struggles, I might offer them a mirror. One that reflects not judgment, but insight, if they should choose to look.

4.1 The Inner Child of a Self-Absorbed Person

I learned early
that my tears annoyed you.
So I swallowed them whole,
like bitter seeds.

I grew small in the corners,
a shadow of myself,
trying to earn a glance,
a touch,
a word that meant I mattered.

But silence grew louder than my laughter.
So I made masks from scraps of attention,
wore them until they felt like skin,
and called it "me."

Inside, I still whisper:
Do you see me yet?
Do you see me?

Children are naturally keen observers of their caregivers - they have to be, as their survival and well-being depend on having their needs met. Mirror neurons play a crucial role in this early development, particularly in learning and social understanding. Located in the same regions of the brain that control action and perception, mirror neurons are activated when we observe someone acting. These neurons enable children to learn through imitation, interpret the actions and intentions of others, and begin developing empathy.

Because of mirror neurons, children learn to smile when they see someone smiling, to respond when they witness someone crying, and to seek connection through shared emotional cues. But when a caregiver is self-centred or emotionally unavailable, the child learns to mirror that self-centeredness or emotional distance. If the caregiver is neglectful or abusive, the child adapts by becoming hyper-vigilant, constantly monitoring their environment to anticipate the caregiver's next move. This survival strategy makes them highly attuned to others' needs, often at the cost of their own. They become skilled at reading emotional cues, pleasing others to gain attention, affection, or to ensure their basic needs are met.

People give meaning to their life experiences through the lens of their perception. The brain interprets information from the environment not only through the filter of past experiences, but also through innate temperament and personality traits. The meaning we assign to our experiences manifests as thoughts that, in turn, shape our reality.

This helps explain why not all children raised in dysfunctional home environments develop self-absorption traits. Even when siblings grow up in the same household, their internal responses to pain and adversity can differ dramatically. Some children may surrender to their circumstances, becoming passive or chronically unhappy. Others might overcompensate by seeking control or achievement, while some learn to avoid conflict altogether. Each child adapts in their way, trying to survive and make sense of their emotional world. Most self-absorbed individuals carry within them a deeply wounded inner child, often shaped by an unstable and emotionally unsafe home environment.

Enmeshment is a common dynamic in such families, particularly when one or both parents exhibit self-absorption traits. In these systems, a lack of healthy differentiation leads to emotional dependency. Instead of fostering relationships grounded in mutuality, respect, and empathy, the dominant parent exerts excessive control, viewing their children as extensions of themselves rather than as separate individuals. In enmeshed families, loyalty is prized above all else, while outsiders are viewed with suspicion and often targeted for criticism; parents demand unwavering obedience, and when it's not given, the child is usually met with mistreatment: devaluation, ridicule, gaslighting, shaming, and isolation.

The psychological effects of enmeshment and abuse are deep and enduring. The child internalizes limiting beliefs about themselves, developing a fragile or distorted sense of identity. They learn that their needs are secondary to those of the family, and are burdened with the pressure of meeting the unrealistic expectations of the abusive parent. Over time, the inner child becomes emotionally depleted, constantly on guard, hypervigilant, and ready to defend against harm.

These tensions intensify in enmeshed families where dynamics are dominated by self-absorption traits when parents show clear favouritism toward one child while expressing disappointment or criticism toward another. In such environments, love becomes conditional and unevenly distributed, granted only to those who meet the parents' unspoken needs for admiration, compliance, or performance. Affection is no longer a birthright, but a reward for aligning with the parent's idealized image of how a child should be.

When parental love is weaponized in this way, competition is sown between siblings. One child may be idealized, treated as special, superior, or entitled, while another may be criticized, dismissed, or emotionally sidelined. This dynamic breeds confusion, shame, and insecurity in the child who is devalued, and it can distort the self-perception of the one who is elevated. Over time, children in both roles may internalize their assigned identities:

- one developing a sense of superiority, internalizing their parents' entitlement. They come to view others as extensions of themselves, and their relationships take on a transactional quality, marked by control, conditionality, and an inability to empathize or genuinely recognize the needs and boundaries of others;

- the other develops a chronic sense of dependency, longing for validation, compliance, and silencing their own needs to accommodate those of others.

In time, these rigid dynamics become emotionally suffocating, as the black-and-white thinking often prevails in those who display a sense of superiority. Conversations are rarely open-ended explorations; they are battlegrounds for dominance, where curiosity is replaced by certainty and emotional attunement gives way to unsolicited advice. The need to be "right" often overshadows the need to connect. Emotional hierarchy persists into adulthood, with one person assuming the role of the perpetual authority.

In more severe cases, the child may experience not only emotional neglect but also physical abuse. The greater the terror, neglect, or control inflicted, the more emotionally dysregulated the child becomes. Some children respond with hyperarousal, crying uncontrollably, yelling, screaming, hitting, kicking, throwing objects, slamming doors, biting, or erupting in explosive outbursts. Others respond with hypoarousal, shutting down entirely to protect themselves. These children learn to hide their emotions, disconnect from their bodies, and silence their pain. Over time, the suppression of negative emotions, used as a coping mechanism, can also dampen their capacity for joy. They may begin to feel numb, like an empty shell moving through life, disconnected from any sense of vitality or inner aliveness.

Other people who display self-absorbed traits were raised by parents who failed to set boundaries or provide consistent discipline. As a result, their inner child did not learn essential social and emotional skills, such as patience, responsibility, or respect for others' needs. When faced with resistance, they often reacted with tantrums, manipulation, or emotional withdrawal, responses that were either ignored or enabled by caregivers. These parents may have modelled similar behaviour themselves, reinforcing a belief system rooted in entitlement, exceptionalism, and a lack of accountability. Over time, the child internalized the idea that their desires should be prioritized above all else and that others existed primarily to serve or reflect their needs.

Having overprotective parents is another factor that can contribute to the development of narcissistic traits. Although the overprotective and overgiving parts of these parents often stem from good intentions, wanting to give their children the life they never had, their excessive involvement can create deep-seated insecurities. The child becomes emotionally and practically dependent on others, lacking the confidence and skills to navigate challenges independently.

Often referred to as "*helicopter parents*," these caregivers tend to sacrifice their own needs to constantly monitor and manage their child's life. They intervene in every difficulty, shielding the child from failure and discomfort, thereby robbing them of the chance to develop resilience, problem-solving abilities, and emotional regulation. To boost their child's self-esteem, these parents may exaggerate accomplishments and avoid offering constructive feedback, fearing it could damage their child's fragile sense of self.

As a result, the inner child grows up without learning how to face disappointment or tolerate frustration. They expect others to accommodate them, often becoming emotionally dysregulated when their needs aren't instantly met. Their self-esteem becomes externally anchored, shaped not by a solid inner foundation but by how others perceive them, especially in terms of success or failure. In adulthood, this can manifest as self-absorption, entitlement, and a fear of vulnerability masked by grandiosity or perfectionism.

Despite being part of a family, when the very people who are meant to protect and nurture them become the source of harm, children are left feeling lost and deeply confused. The home, supposed to be a place of safety, becomes unpredictable, even dangerous. When a child is remote-controlled by the mind, needs, and expectations of their caregivers, they lose connection with their inner world. To survive, they feel compelled to establish some sense of control, however fragile, over their environment, emotions, and the way they are perceived by others.

In this effort to gain safety and approval, they often suppress or disown parts of themselves. Vulnerability, in such an environment, becomes a threat, something that can be used against them. So, they learn to mask it, presenting a version of themselves that is more acceptable, more pleasing, or more invisible, depending on what the situation demands. Over time, this protective adaptation can harden into a false self, leaving the inner child unseen, unheard, and aching for connection.

Regardless of whether the inner child of a self-absorbed person experienced abuse, neglect, or overprotection, they often internalize a set of maladaptive beliefs about themselves. Deep down, this inner child believes they are not good enough, defective, inadequate, incompetent, and unlovable. These core beliefs create ongoing emotional turmoil. The inner child feels vulnerable, ashamed, anxious, and chronically unsafe. They are conditioned to expect rejection, humiliation, and control from others. This internal landscape is marked by a persistent sense of emptiness, dissatisfaction, and longing.

In response to these painful emotions: jealousy, shame, unworthiness, protective parts emerge. These parts carry the burden of trying to give the inner child what they never received from their caregivers: validation, approval, safety, and love. Yet, in doing so, they often adopt rigid, controlling, or self-centred behaviours, hoping to soothe the wounded inner child through external means. What begins as a survival strategy becomes an ingrained pattern that affects not only the self-absorbed person but everyone in their emotional orbit.

To cope with the void left by the absence of love and emotional attunement from their caregivers, the inner child begins to retreat into fantasy. They imagine idealized versions of love, power, greatness, success, beauty, and brilliance, realms where they are finally seen, celebrated, and safe. These fantasies become cherished companions, offering comfort, relief, and a sense of purpose that their external world cannot provide.

Over time, these fantasies evolve into the seeds of their protective parts - constructed identities designed to shield the inner child from further pain. As these parts grow stronger, the inner child begins to lose touch with reality. The fantasy world becomes more compelling than the real one, creating a growing disconnection from their Self. The farther they drift from the Self, the harder it becomes to face vulnerability, uncertainty, and emotional intimacy without the armour of illusion.

From my own lived experience - as a survivor of abuse from self-absorbed people and as a mental health professional, who has come to support both survivors and a few individuals with self-absorption traits - I've come to understand that dominant protective parts often emerge early in childhood. The earlier these parts develop, the more deeply ingrained they become, making them harder to heal. When the inner child endures chronic abuse, neglect, or control, more protective parts are forced to surface as survival mechanisms. Each new wound gives rise to another layer of defence, gradually burying the child's vulnerability beneath masks of entitlement, detachment, or superiority.

Like anyone who has experienced abuse, self-absorbed individuals struggle with cognitive dissonance - a persistent conflict between their protective parts and their wounded inner child. While their protective parts may be hypervigilant and aware of the risk of further harm, the inner child remains emotionally tethered to the hope of receiving the love, validation, and approval they never had. The love of their inner child is like an obsessive-compulsive attachment to romantic partners. The fantasy of being loved by someone soothes their pain, validates self-worth, and can cause withdrawal symptoms when the relationship ends or shifts, causing significant disruption in one's emotional, social, or occupational life.

This unmet longing for love often compels them to maintain contact with their abusive parents and other family members, reenacting the trauma in hopes of rewriting the outcome. In these moments, the inner child's yearning tends to override the protective parts, leaving them sometimes powerless to the abuse of their parents and siblings. I've witnessed this inner child most vulnerable and emotionally dysregulated within the confines of their home environment, where old wounds are easily reopened.

Offering love to the wounded inner child of a self-absorbed person doesn't help them feel lovable. The belief that they are unlovable runs deep; it is ingrained, persistent, and resistant. No one can make us feel something we are not willing or ready to feel. The protective parts of this inner child are highly skeptical, even dismissive, of any evidence that someone truly cares for them. To them, love feels like a closed chapter; something they once hoped for, but eventually abandoned as impossible. Their reactions are shaped by a painful awareness of the manipulative strategies they've developed to survive, and a haunting fear that others might one day use similar strategies against their inner child. These protective parts allow their inner child to enjoy the fantasy of finding love, but continue to whisper their opinions in their ears to ensure that there is no risk of potential hurt.

Under certain conditions, the inner child's protective parts can relax when they don't feel vulnerable, threatened, or exposed. In those rare moments, their inner child may appear joyful, kind, and vibrant. These moments reveal the raw emotions in their eyes, as they cling to moments of warmth and hope. An inner child who wants to be loved. It is only in such moments that the victims can see them capable of expressing genuine emotional and compassionate empathy. These glimpses of who they truly are can be deeply moving, creating hope and emotional whiplash for those close to them. The victim may begin to question their perception of abuse or cling to the belief that change is possible, yearning to connect more often with this seemingly loving and open part of the person. Unfortunately, these moments are often short-lived. Their protective parts, ever hypervigilant, quickly resurface, afraid that any softness or vulnerability might expose the inner child to further harm. And so, the cycle continues, with tenderness giving way once again to defence, denial, and control.

Self-love is the foundation of any healthy relationship. Before we can relate to others in a meaningful way, we must first build a respectful, compassionate relationship with ourselves. When we have a strong sense of self-worth and inner stability, we are more likely to form connections with people who reflect those same values; people who don't rely on others to define their identity.

Through my lived experiences, I've come to realize that I am not truly loving my inner child if I allow others to mistreat her. Protecting her is an act of self-respect. In the same way, no matter how much love is offered to the inner child of a self-absorbed person, they cannot receive it. Until they learn to see themselves as worthy, until they choose to meet their wounds with honesty and care, the love of others will always feel out of reach, questioned, or dismissed. To experience true love, they must unlearn self-hate, release the insecurities and shame that others have projected onto them, and stop hurting other people. Without this inner transformation, they will continue to sabotage the very relationships they long for, repeating a cycle of heartbreak and disconnection.

My hands were always reaching for love,

for warmth,
for the kind of safety that never came.

When it didn't arrive,
I built castles of self-importance,
hoping their towers
would make you look up at me.

But even the tallest walls
cannot fill a hollow belly.
The hunger still gnaws,
a child pounding on the inside of the chest,
crying for what was never fed.

All the praise in the world
cannot quiet that child.
The child only ever wanted
to be held.

4.2 The "In Control" Protector

I hold the reins tight.
Every step, every glance, every word
I steer them all,
so the chaos never spills
into the fragile corners inside.

I measure, I plan, I correct.
Mistakes are dangers.
Failure is an enemy.
I am tireless,
because if I falter,
everything could crumble.

I am the armor,
the walls, the unyielding line.
No one sees the trembling beneath,
and if they did,
they would leave.

There comes a pivotal moment in the life of a traumatized inner child when they must choose, consciously or not, whether to keep their heart open to love or close it off entirely. From this turning point, when the child chooses to close their heart off, a powerful "in control" protective part often emerges. This part arises from the fierce need to reject vulnerability in every interpersonal relationship the inner child encounters. In the mind of this protector, love is synonymous with pain, something dangerous and not to be trusted. Therefore, it must be avoided or dismissed at all costs.

The belief that no one can be trusted doesn't form in a vacuum. It is born from one or more deeply traumatic experiences, moments when the child couldn't make sense of what was happening and, instead of being met with compassion or comfort, was left exposed, invalidated, or betrayed. Unable to express their needs safely, the child's nervous system shuts down the possibility of trust, replacing it with hypervigilance and a need for control. Over time, this protector becomes not just a shield, but a barrier between the inner child and the love they so desperately crave.

> Love, where the hell are you?
> You're the only balm
> for this wound inside.
> And still,
> I don't believe
> you exist.

This is one of the earliest protective parts to emerge in self-absorbed individuals. In my mind's eye, I see it as a shield, designed to be unbreakable. In the reality this part constructs, people are no longer seen as human beings but as objects: tools to be used, controlled, and discarded at will.

When this shield is formed, it gives rise to fantasies, illusions of success, power, brilliance, revenge, and romantic idealism that help the inner child reject the painful truths of their reality. These fantasies become the scaffolding for all the other protective parts that follow. The moment these fantasies take root is also the moment they begin to disconnect from their Self.

The "in control" protector plays a central role. Without its constant effort to keep the inner child emotionally distant, from themselves and others, all the other protectors would struggle to fulfill their roles. In return, this part depends on the others to keep the shield alive. Whenever the other protective parts craft dishonest narratives, deny vulnerability, or inflate grandiosity, the shield grows stronger. Sadly, this only leaves the inner child more disconnected, dependent on fantasy, and starved of real love.

This protector is often easy to spot in real life. It presents as physical presence paired with emotional absence. Once the victim is "secured" by the charming chameleon protector, the "in control" part becomes dominant, offering little to no empathy or support.

If any protector begins to evolve, attempting to adopt new tools or drop the old strategies, the others often resist. Change means admitting manipulation, dishonesty, and the desire to dominate. But ultimately, no shift is possible without the permission of the "in control" part, because all protectors emerged the moment the child began fantasizing as a way to regain control. However, I consider that the ultimate decision to bring positive changes in their lives belongs to the inner child. These changes may come only after their inner child acknowledges the destructive impact of their protective parts'decisions on their lives, is saturated by them, and they see glimpses of the life they could have when being connected to their Self.

Although this part is built from a conscious decision to protect the inner child from emotional pain, its influence can intensify unconsciously based on external triggers. In situations that echo past shame or guilt, the protector may activate dissociation, derealization, or depersonalization, defense mechanisms that create emotional and even physical numbness.

I once saw this firsthand with my father. One night, he poured hot soup over his hands and didn't even notice. By the time I took the bowl from him, he was still unaware of the pain. It took him several moments to reorient to the present. That was a brief episode of dissociation, but for some, these episodes can last for days or weeks, especially after contact with their childhood environments or family members. In these states, reality may feel altered, people may seem like characters from an old "movie," and emotional connection is impossible.

Despite all this, there *are* rare moments when this protector relaxes, when it isn't triggered, and feels safe. These windows of trust may open:

- With a victim who mirrors the same kind of wounds as their own inner child.

- With a therapist, *if* the individual begins to trust and *if* the other protectors are willing to adopt new strategies.

In these moments, their inner child becomes accessible, grounded, joyful, kind, full of love. But the level of control exerted by the "in control" protector varies from person to person. Unlike other protectors that may develop some level of self-awareness, this one often refuses to acknowledge its own motives, not even in private reflection.Their typical response is to numb the emotions of their inner child. *"If I feel too much, my inner child will be overwhelmed,"* this part reasons. *"So I must shut the system down.* This explains why self-absorbed individuals may deny being self-absorbed not just to others, but to themselves as well.

When something triggers old wounds, shame, rejection, or feelings of inadequacy, this protector springs into action. It recruits "firefighters" to restore control: binge eating, casual sex, substance use. It also shows up when asked to show empathy or take accountability. A simple request to put themselves in other people's shoes can catch this protector off guard. Even a fleeting moment of acknowledgment could awaken the inner child's suppressed guilt and shame." In such moments, the victim may briefly witness the expressions of other protective parts, rage, guilt, shame, or even a contemptuous smirk, flashing across their face in a matter of minutes.

Often, this response shows up on their face, a blank, confused expression, as the protector quickly evaluates which mask to put on next. Most of the time, it's either the manipulative or chameleon protector who steps forward to handle the situation.

A spark touches old wounds
shame, rejection, the hollow ache.
The protector rises, sharp and swift,
summoning its fire:
binge, escape, numbness, indulgence.

A simple question, a hint of empathy,
and the mask falters.
A flicker of guilt, a shadow of rage,
a smirk, a flash
all in the mirror of the face.

Blank eyes scan, calculating,
which mask to wear next:
manipulator, chameleon,
anything to keep the child inside
hidden, safe...
for now.

4.3 The Chameleon Protector

Born in a room of unspoken rules,
a soft soul learned to bend and sway.
Shadows whispered, *be what is wanted,*
and the mask became the safest way.

Eyes grew sharp, reading the air,
not for truth, but for survival.
Every smile, every tilt of voice,
a code to crack, a stage for revival.

The chameleon weaves colors of safety,
shifting tones to match the crowd.
Authenticity locked behind the curtain,
while applause for the mask grew loud.

Yet beneath the costumes and borrowed skin,
still lives a longing, fierce and true:
to stand unpainted, unafraid,
and be loved for simply being *you.*

The chameleon protective part is typically the first one the victim encounters. It corresponds to the *love bombing* phase in the abuse cycle with self-absorbed people, and its primary role is to create an image that aligns with the environment and serves the deeper agenda of the manipulative protective part. It is also the protector who shows up at a job interview or any other social situation. This part first emerges early in life, often during childhood, when the inner child begins to closely observe their caregivers' behavior in order to survive. By mirroring what their parents wanted to see, the child learns to adapt, shape-shift, and become whoever they need to be to stay safe, gain attention, and have their basic needs met. Since then, this part has remained highly active, constantly studying people's body language, emotional cues, and psychological patterns to refine its performance. It develops a sharp cognitive empathy, not to build authentic connection, but to better anticipate what others want and to gain approval, power, or control.

Just as a chess player prepares for a match- reviewing openings, analyzing past games, and mentally and physically conditioning themselves - this protective part activates well before an encounter the manipulative part deems important. It meticulously gathers information about the new target, studying their interests, behaviors, and emotional patterns to determine the most effective approach. The goal is to craft a striking first impression, one powerful enough to ensure they won't simply blend into the crowd, but instead become unforgettable.

At the beginning of the relationship, the chameleon protective part carefully studies the potential victim, eager to uncover their values, beliefs, past experiences, aspirations, and insecurities. Based on these observations, it constructs and performs an ideal persona, one that not only reflects the victim's own story and values but also embodies everything the victim hopes to find in a partner: confidence, humor, emotional and financial stability, and above all, reliability.

To attract the type of victim they want, this part is willing to undergo noticeable changes - losing weight, altering their clothing style, changing their hairstyle, adjusting their tone of voice, and modifying their verbal and facial expressions. This part is skilled at displaying a range of expressions: warmth, shyness, flirtation, charm, confidence.

If you suspect you're in a relationship with someone who exhibits self-absorption traits, take a closer look at the photos they shared with you early on, especially during the love bombing phase. You might notice facial expressions that radiate warmth, kindness, and attentiveness, expressions that have likely faded or disappeared over time. These early images often reflect the carefully crafted persona of the chameleon protective part. This false image is also evident on their social media: frequent selfies, flashy clothing, heavy makeup, old photos from when they appeared younger or slimmer, or heavily edited pictures designed to conceal perceived flaws. Every detail is curated to maintain the illusion of perfection and to reinforce the identity they want others to see.

At the beginning of a relationship, the chameleon protective part strategically uses flattery to make their victim feel special and admired, with the hidden hope that this behavior will be mirrored back. They might say things like: *"You're so kindhearted," "You're truly special," "You deserve to be loved," "You are a great boss*" or "*You matter more than....*" These compliments aren't spontaneous expressions of genuine affection, they are calculated moves designed to build trust and attachment.

To reinforce the illusion of emotional availability and reliability, this part may ask for the victim's opinion before making shared decisions, show up during a few moments of need to appear dependable, express interest in meeting their friends and family, and even cry during emotional movies. All of these gestures serve to strengthen the illusion that they are emotionally present, caring, and trustworthy, when, in fact, it's a carefully rehearsed act.

Purposefully, this part avoids drawing attention to the victim's insecurities, acting as though they haven't even noticed them. However, every detail, every vulnerability quietly shared or subtly revealed, is carefully recorded and stored like a file, to be handed off to the manipulative protective part later. Once trust and emotional attachment have been established, those insecurities become tools, leverage used to gain control and power over the victim when the dynamic begins to shift from idealization to devaluation.

When their potential victim begins to open up and embrace vulnerability, the chameleon part mirrors that vulnerability, often through stories. In my work with self-absorbed people, I have noticed that the chameleon protective part hyperfocuses on their inner child's struggles to attract empathy and compassion. The work has never gone beyond this phase, as other protective parts, but especially the manipulative one, don't want to become the focus of these therapeutic conversations. To reflect vulnerability, this part also chooses to shift focus to the struggles of a close friend or relative, presenting those stories to elicit sympathy by association with these people.

A more educated chameleon protective part often leans into creating a false image of humility, especially at the beginning of a relationship. This pseudo-humility is a calculated strategy designed to lower suspicion by avoiding the appearance of always blaming others for past failures. Through triangulation, this part shares stories about previous relationships, friends and family members, often exaggerating their faults while selectively admitting to their own mistakes. However, when they do take responsibility, it is carefully measured, minimized and reframed in a way that still protects their image.

To further impress their potential victim, this part frequently shares false stories of their charity and selflessness, presenting them as someone deeply kind and generous. These narratives often conclude with the inner child cast as the unrecognized or underappreciated giver, subtly evoking the victim's compassion or sympathy. Other times, the chameleon part presents the inner child as someone who doesn't care about recognition, claiming they never needed external validation, another performance meant to reinforce the illusion of emotional maturity and strength, while keeping the victim emotionally engaged and admiring.

Hypocrisy is another defining trait of the chameleon protective part, whose primary focus is maintaining a positive image of the inner child. While this part often downplays or minimizes the harmful actions of the inner child or other protective parts, it eagerly absorbs praise and recognition from others. When the victim offers admiration or validation, the chameleon part feels a surge of satisfaction. This moment of external affirmation serves as a temporary boost to the inner child's fragile self-esteem. Internally, the inner child affirms this image with a quiet, self-soothing reassurance: *"That's who I am."* In these fleeting moments, the illusion of worthiness becomes their reality, at least for a little while.

Lies and triangulation are also used to impress their victim, who might not be able to detect them until after their relationship ended.

> They spoke in webs of words,
> twisting truths,
> weaving lies into patterns I couldn't see.
>
> A shadow play of smiles and stories,
> triangles drawn in air,
> each angle designed to ensnare.
>
> I only recognize it now,
> after the chapters closed,
> the hidden lines finally clear
> the art of control revealed
> when it was too late to touch.

After a period of rest and reflection following the breakup, survivors of narcissistic abuse may begin to uncover answers to previously unanswered questions, especially when they reframe the stories they were told. By mentally replacing the characters in these narratives, patterns begin to emerge. For instance, if the manipulative part criticized the mental health of a former partner (a tactic known as triangulation), they were likely revealing something about their own. If they spoke disapprovingly about a friend who cheated or claimed that infidelity is one of their biggest turn-offs, they were often projecting their own behavior.

From the very beginning of the relationship, the chameleon protective part employs these strategies, boasting about virtues they secretly long to possess in hopes of attracting partners who genuinely embody them. I encourage anyone navigating a new relationship to pay close attention to what people share on social media platforms like Facebook or Instagram. Subtle signs of dishonesty or contradiction often appear in these carefully curated spaces.

> If I bend myself
> to keep your gaze,
> to twist truths
> so you remain intrigued,
>
> I will feel the weight of hate
> pressing inward.

> If I cling to who I am,
> honest and whole,
> the walls I've built may shatter
> and I will crack
> under the strain of wanting and being.

The chameleon protective part may avoid introducing their victim to friends or family altogether, as doing so invites a level of emotional intimacy their inner child isn't ready, or willing to embrace. If they do make introductions, these are calculated and selective. They choose people who reflect the image they want to project, carefully balancing how much vulnerability they're willing to expose and what impression they want to leave on their victim. More often than not, they keep their family at a distance, choosing instead to present friends who appear socially polished and possess qualities they themselves aspire to embody. The deeper the victim falls for this curated reality, the more disoriented and emotionally exposed they become when the manipulative part inevitably begins to surface.

Carrying the role of the chameleon protective part is an exhausting task. Over time, maintaining this carefully crafted persona becomes unsustainable. As the manipulative part secures emotional attachment, effectively gaining power over the victim, the chameleon steps back, becoming less vigilant and eventually deactivated. However, this part can be reactivated if the victim begins to resist, especially when they attempt to end the relationship and no longer respond to the manipulative part's tactics. In such moments, the chameleon may resort to triangulation once again, this time by befriending the victim's friends, family members, coworkers, or even by taking the risk to introduce the victim to their own family. It presents itself as heartbroken and confused, feigning ignorance about the reasons behind the breakup. The goal is to elicit sympathy, hoping those close to the victim will persuade them to return.

The discard of the victim occurs when the chameleon protective part can no longer sustain the illusion, when it runs out of tools to maintain the carefully constructed image, when the manipulative part identifies a new, more desirable target, or when the victim begins to awaken, recognizing the tactics at play and stepping into survivorhood. Another key trigger for discard is when the protectors of their inner child suddenly feel unsafe or overwhelmed, aware that their inner child is at risk becoming vulnerable as the relationship deepens, especially if it moves toward a level of intimacy they are emotionally unprepared to face. In this case, the "in control" part intervenes to protect their inner child from potential future harm. Any one of these reasons can be enough to end the relationship, but often, several converge at once. Sometimes, the discard happens abruptly, leaving the victim with no explanation, no closure. Other times, it is meticulously orchestrated by the chameleon part, designed to make it appear as though ending the relationship was the victim's own decision.

> I cannot walk away from you...
> though sometimes,
> I know I should.
>
> When you desire me,
> I feel valuable, creative, whole.
> I glimpse myself,
> and for a moment,
> I love who I am.
>
> And in that love,
> your love feels even stronger.
> It's a circle I cannot escape
> without you,
> I might never know what love is.

After the relationship ends, the chameleon protective part often steps back, giving the appearance of respecting the victim's decision and offering time and space. This calculated withdrawal is not an act of genuine consideration, but a strategic move, another illusion meant to maintain control while observing the victim's emotional response. The way the victim responds determines whether other protective parts become activated, particularly those that are triggered by rejection. While the chameleon part may re-emerge with warm, appreciative language in an attempt to hoover the victim back in, the other protective parts, driven by shame, rage, or entitlement, often communicate in harsher, more reactive ways, revealing the deeper instability behind the mask.

I wear your shape,
your voice, your moods,
blending in until I disappear.

Every glance, every word,
I shift
to be safe,
to be unseen,
to keep the small one inside
from being crushed.

4.4 The Manipulative Protector

> The chameleon spun the story,
> crafted the illusion,
> and you believed it.
>
> And yet, in that instant,
> I lost respect
> for you,
> for missing the truth
> that I had placed before your eyes.

The inner child of self-absorbed people feels emotions, like any other person. When their inner child got abused over and over again, the "in control" protector started to numb out any pain to be able to survive. The manipulative part is responsible for accessing resources for their inner child to have their needs and wants met.

The manipulative part believes that all people have hidden intentions aimed to control them, they see other people as objects, something that can serve their needs. Consequently, this protective part uses people for money, resources, attention, manipulates people's compassion, dreams, plants little seeds of poison, causing people to doubt their own reality and judgements, violates people's boundaries, isolates their victim away from friends and family, projects their inner child's insecurities onto others, blames other people for whatever is not working well in their lives, uses emotional blackmail to obtain their goals and elicit feelings of fear, guilt and compliance. As the inner child and their protective parts gradually distance themselves from their Self from a young age, they start to gravitate towards the manipulative part, who takes on the leadership position among all of them and coordinates their actions.

This protective part uses slightly different manipulative strategies at different stages of the relationship with their victim.

The presence of this protective part is barely noticeable at the beginning of a relationship as it's hiding behind the chameleon part. However, in tandem with the chameleon part, the manipulative one is responsible for gathering as much information as possible about their future victim to determine if they can serve their own gains and ambitions. The perfect target of the manipulative part has experienced abuse before, is isolated, friendly, kind, altruistic, honest, refrains from judging people, tends to believe that most people can be trusted, is responsible, and diligent. These are some of the most important attributes of their perfect victim. In addition to these traits, this part also searches for other resources, such as money, an upgrade in social status, social network, anything that corresponds with their agenda.

As the manipulative part craves recognition and doesn't like being under the shadow of the chameleon part, the victim receives disguised messages from this part from the beginning of their relationships, signaling their true intentions and testing their victim's ability to detect them. These messages initially seem to fit in the context of their conversations and, most of the time, they get unnoticed for long periods of time. Many survivors of abuse from self-absorbed people understand the true meaning of these messages only after ending the relationship, when they were less emotionally entangled in this connection. Though, if the victim catches them on time and confronts this part, deflection or projection are used to escape that situation.

The manipulative protective part subtly trains future victims on how it expects to be treated, often through passive comparisons or triangulation. It may introduce a third party as an indirect example, using comments like: *"My ex never cooked for me,"*, *"My previous boss always criticized me"*, *"My family doesn't really understand me"* or *"You're not like any of my other friends"*. When this protective part belongs to a parent, it sounds like: *"Your sibling never complains - maybe the problem is you"* or *"I've never had these problems with the other kid(s). You're the only one making drama."* These seemingly casual remarks are loaded with implication, planting the seed of obligation, guilt, or pressure in the listener - shaping their behavior to meet the part's unspoken needs. Once these goals are achieved, the manipulative part demands their victim to continue complimenting them, even if their behavior becomes abusive.

In the first stages of a relationship, the manipulative part plays the victim role in a subtle way, appealing for their altruism to have them do things for them. Over time, the victim is expected to step in and help every time is needed. Then, the expectation becomes a must. They may also try to trap the victim by proposing team work on projects that benefit only them, but the victim ends up doing all the work. This part uses *bargaining tactics* to manipulate others into giving them what they want. To achieve this goal, this protective part doesn't hesitate making these kinds of requests in the name of love: *"If you are a good child, you do this for me"*, *"Don't you love me?"*, *"Be the bigger person - let this go and I'll make it up to you"* or *"If you just stop bringing up the past, I'll try to be nicer moving forward."*

Even if this protective part claims wanting to do things equally, it is never in their intention to fulfill their promise.

As the relationship evolves, the manipulative part starts to cross the boundaries of their victim. They create rules and expectations that benefit themselves and then claim that their victim agreed with them. Oftentimes, they change the rules if they no longer serve them and, if exposed, this part brings the chameleon part in this mind game to create the illusion of fairness or uses other control tactics to intimidate others into compliance.

Partner: *"You said you were okay with me needing space. Now you're mad when I don't answer your texts for hours?"*

You: *"I said I understood you were busy. That's different from disappearing without explanation."*

Partner: *"You're always changing the story. It's impossible to please you."*

Parent: *"I just want peace in this family. If I'm the problem, fine-I'll stay away."*

(Later, they call another sibling:)

Parent: *"She's been so cold lately. I don't know what I did to deserve this, but I guess she's turned into one of those toxic types who cut off their family."*

Guilt-tripping is a form of emotional manipulation that elicits feelings of guilt in their victim if they try to question their sovereignty. It preys on the victim's sense of responsibility toward other aspects of their lives, making them feel guilty for wanting to spend time with their children, friends, or investing in their passions by blaming them for not spending time with them, not paying attention to their needs, or for not doing enough to help. The reason behind this tactic is to isolate their victims from other people and reduce the likelihood of having outside interference in the dynamic between them.

Another manipulative strategy used by this protective part is gaslighting. Gaslighting is a deliberate form of emotional abuse that causes victims to question their reality, memories, and sanity. Many victims might not even be aware of it until the manipulative part establishes control over them and, by that time, the victim starts to blame themselves for not giving enough to make their relationship work. This protective part dismisses evidence that demonstrates their victim's dedication and love and purposely recalls situations when their victim tried to set boundaries and declined to help. The use of gaslighting stems from the manipulative part's inability to acknowledge their victim's words and actions, and a deep desire to gain control over them. Some examples of gaslighting are: *"You are imagining this"*, *"You misunderstand what I've said"*, *"I don't know what you are talking about"*, *"You are too sensitive"*, *"You don't know what you are talking about"*, *"You have a bad memory"*, *"I didn't say that..."*, *"That never happened"*, *"You are crazy"*.

Projection is another manipulative strategy used by this protective part. Whenever a situation triggers the memories of their inner child that caused them to feel insecure, ashamed, inferior, this protective part steps in to shift the responsibility and blame from them onto their victim. Accusations of cheating, lying, being angry, jealous, a narcissist, are shouted out to intimidate their partner and provoke a corrosive reaction in their self-esteem.

> Most loneliness
> is a quiet sting,
> peering into fractured mirrors
> of my own sorrow,
> hoping, for a fleeting moment,
> to find someone else
> to blame the ache on.

Gaslighting and projection are insidious tactics that cause emotional abuse and create conflict among the victim's inner child and their protective parts, a conflict that is known as cognitive dissonance. It is important to know that both the chameleon part and the manipulative one use projection, the difference between their use of this strategy lies in their intention. While the chameleon part uses triangulation to project their insecurities onto others to impress their new potential victim, the manipulative one uses projection to create insecurities and control their "already" victim.

Triangulation is often used in enmeshed families. It is a passive-aggressive form of communication that goes through a third-party to convey a message to the target. Unlike the chameleon part, who uses this strategy at the onset of the relationship to make their victim feel special, the manipulative one makes use of it to compare their victim to a previous partner or a family member. They highlight how well treated they have been by someone else to create competition, shame, erode the victim's confidence, and isolate them from others. At times, triangulation is used when discarding their victim, as the manipulative protective part wants to cause shame and gain satisfaction by involving a third party, who views that opportunity like a vulture drawn to roadkill.

Most of the time, when we begin a relationship, we feel safe, unaware that the other person sees us as competitors, potential threats for their insecure inner child. We may share with them intimate experiences that disclose some of our insecurities and we may not notice from the beginning the shield that is built around their inner child. Yet, we don't foresee that they will use those moments of vulnerability as psychological ammunition. Once the manipulative part is certain that emotional attachment has been created between them and the victim, the file containing the victim's insecurities gets opened. With a condescending tone of voice, they put their victim down to gain control over them. The information that was shared by the victim in a moment of vulnerability and that was meant to bring emotional connection is perceived by this protective part as insecurity. This protective part will never make such a decision that makes their inner child vulnerable to harm. Sometimes, this part uses sensitive information about their victim in front of others that may sound like an inside joke. If confronted, the chameleon part denies the malicious meaning of their comment or even claims that they make a humorous joke, nothing to be offended of.

To increase their level of control over their victim, the manipulative part makes use of convincing narratives to have them give up on their jobs, dreams, everything that brings stability into their lives. If this approach doesn't work, this part uses other tactics to accomplish their plan, such as sabotaging their victim's ability to go to work, study, and meet with their friends or family members. For example, this part may take the risk of embarrassing the victim in front of their friends, complaining about their behaviors, and creating reasons to keep their victim at home when planning to meet with people they care about, hoping that their victim will choose them against their friends afterwards. The more isolated their victim is, the more power this part has over them.

The manipulative protector of a self-absorbed person can skillfully weave spirituality into their control tactics, using it as both a shield and a weapon. With the help of the grandiose protector, who presents themselves as enlightened, morally superior, or uniquely connected to divine wisdom, creating an aura of unquestionable authority, the spiritual language of the manipulative protector becomes a tool to justify their behavior, insisting that their actions are "*for your highest good*" or that any resistance is a sign you are "*not ready to ascend*" or "s*till trapped in ego.*" They might selectively quote sacred texts, reinterpret mystical concepts, or claim to receive special guidance that conveniently aligns with their own desires. In this way, spirituality is stripped of its authentic power to connect and heal, and instead is distorted into a framework where questioning them equates to questioning truth itself.

When the chameleon protective part starts to feel tired and loses their convincing power, the manipulative part may use creative manipulative ways to maintain control over their victim. If their victim mirrors some of their wounds and their relationship has the potential to evolve, this manipulative part shares pieces of information related to the wounds of their inner child, the purpose being to gain compassion and empathy that are to be used in order to manipulate the victim into staying in this relationship.

The silent treatment is a form of emotional abuse that creates a lot of anxiety in victims, as they start questioning themselves, wondering if they have done something to cause that reaction. It encompasses the purpose of all their other manipulative tactics without saying any words. What is less known though is that this strategy is also used after a situation that caused a significant emotional destabilization that had a ripple effect on all the protective parts of this deeply wounded inner child. This tactic masks the need of all these parts to recollect and strategize their next moves. The next move could come from any of their protective parts, depending on the desired outcome of the manipulative part.

When there is enough evidence that reflects full control over their victim, this protective part may want to initiate their victim into manipulating others. The victim's ability to recognize this manipulative tactic and the potential outcomes that come from becoming complacent with them can change this game, as resistance can lead to the victim's discard immediately. This is a very tricky tactic that reveals the true nature of this protective part who not only doesn't want to be recognized, but is expecting full obedience from their victim.

After the discard, or even when the victim finds the strength to walk away, a period of apparent rest often follows. It feels like relief, as if the storm has finally passed. Yet this peace is only an illusion. Sooner or later, the manipulative protective part re-emerges, slipping quietly back into the victim's life, reminding them of old fears, doubts, and longings. This move is part of the game played by their manipulative part, which is similar to how a cat plays with the mouse, wanting to tire them out before killing it. The manipulative part is aware that this illusion causes confusion to the victim because the victim didn't have enough time to emotionally detach from them and still struggles with cognitive dissonance. If their victim is slow in their recovery, lethargic, doesn't see the illusion and returns to them, the victim can easily fall into this trap, making their inner child feel wanted and loved again. When the manipulation is successful, this protective part feels more power over their victim. It may not help in your recovery process, but the manipulative part gains some respect for their victim only after the victim breaks this cycle.

The return of the manipulative part is not with apologies and humbleness. Most of the time, this part is unable to acknowledge their harming actions. However, there are times when the victim's comments penetrate the shield built by the manipulative part, triggering the emotions of their inner child. In those short moments, the victim can see the face of shame. Their narrative is scriptic, focused on their reflections and how special their victim is, and it lacks accountability for their own hurtful actions.

Many survivors of narcissistic abuse expect apologies from their perpetrators. Only a few of them may cleverly make use of apologies to hoover their victim again. Most of the time, the apology never comes, because it destroys the image of their inner child. The narrative of the chameleon protective part following the break up of their relationship focuses on soothing their inner child by constructing a victim image for themselves while painting their victim as the villain. The narrative for their inner child sounds like: *"She/he doesn't know what she/he lost"*, *"Too bad, they' ve lost my attention"*, *"There are two people in a relationship and I can't do anything if the other one doesn't want to work on making the relationship work"*, or *"It hasn't been easy for me to handle break-ups; it's not healthy for me to receive hope each time when we get together and then get disappointed when we break up again"*.

This part is in charge of creating smear campaigns by spreading lies to the victim's family, friends, coworkers and depicting their victim as an impostor, cruel and unavailable person, who mistreated them. The smear campaigns start even before the discard phase to strategically discredit their victim.

> If I break apart,
> at least you cannot reach me.
> I will vanish into myself,
> unaware, uncaring,
> as if you do not exist.

4.5 The Grandiose Protector

> I sit above the chaos,
> king of careful steps and polished smiles.
> Every word I speak
> is a shield,
> every gesture a crown.
>
> I cannot falter,
> cannot show the cracks beneath the gold.
> My grandeur keeps the world at bay,
> the fragile child inside
> hidden behind walls of pride.
>
> No one must see
> how small I truly feel,
> so I reign, flawless and untouchable,
> while the heart within waits silently.

This grandiose protective part usually emerges when the inner child, chronically deprived of validation, recognition, or consistent emotional presence, begins to fantasize about being powerful, admired, and exceptional. These fantasies serve as a psychological escape from the crushing weight of unmet needs and internalized shame. When the child is forced to meet unrealistic expectations or is only praised for performing, achieving, or pleasing, a split occurs: the child's authentic self, burdened by rejection and inadequacy, retreats into exile, while the grandiose protector steps forward to compensate.

Because the inner child longs to feel special, seen, and valuable, this protector builds an idealized image around them marked by superiority and uniqueness. It is not seeking connection, but elevation.

The grandiose part of self-absorbed people whose inner child barely heard the word "no", was excused from basic responsibilities, and didn't face consequences after breaking rules, emerged early in their life, holding a developed sense of entitlement. Consequently, this protective part lacks appreciation for what it was given to them, believes that they must receive everything they want, doesn't learn to take accountability for their actions, and sees themselves as receivers, but not givers. When not getting their own way, this protective part is unable to tolerate frustration and triggers the revengeful firefighter.

In social situations, the grandiose part instinctively steers attention toward itself, believing that admiration and external validation can repair the deep wounds of worthlessness carried by the inner child. To this part, other people become mirrors, not companions, reflectors of status, beauty, talent, intelligence, or success.

This part's narratives are almost always centered around enhancement of the false self: stories of achievement, talent, popularity, opulence, or perceived superiority. The primary goal is to manufacture admiration that the child was once denied. As a result, this part often pursues leadership roles, accolades, or status symbols, not for genuine self-expression or fulfillment, but to secure external proof that the inner child is valuable, lovable, and "better than."

The grandiose part sees life as a constant competition. Relationships become arenas where dominance must be asserted, and others are unconsciously cast as rivals, critics, or supporters of the image they are trying to maintain. This competitiveness is not fueled by arrogance alone, but by fear: if they are not the best, they are no one. If they are not admired, they are invisible. There is no room for nuance or complexity. People are either "good" or "bad," "right" or "wrong," "winners" or "losers." This black-and-white thinking mirrors the child's early experiences of parental favoritism or conditional love, where survival meant competing with others for affection and significance.

When the grandiose part succeeds in receiving praise, admiration, or external validation, the inner child feels temporarily soothed, even euphoric. In those moments, the part believes it has done its job: it has proven the child is lovable. But when it fails, when a goal is missed, admiration is withheld, or criticism is received, the fragile illusion collapses. The inner child, still carrying a negative self-perception, is retraumatized. This can lead to sudden emotional shifts: elation followed by despair, confidence followed by shame, joy followed by rage or anxiety.

These oscillations reflect the internal tug-of-war between the grandiose protector's inflated self-image and the exiled child's buried wounds of unworthiness.

The grandiose protector does not look the same in everyone. In some, especially vulnerable self-absorbed people, it operates covertly, masked in self-pity, martyrdom, or subtle resentment: *"I've worked just as hard, but I never get recognized," "Success isn't for people like me," "It's not fair - I do everything right and still get nowhere."* These statements carry a hidden entitlement - the belief that recognition is owed, but unjustly withheld.

In others, especially overt self-absorbed people, the grandiose part is bold and unfiltered: *"Success comes naturally to me. I'm built differently," "I deserve more than most people - I'm simply more talented,"* or *"People like me are meant to be at the top."* The underlying hunger is the same; both versions crave admiration, respect, and proof that they matter.

In truth, neither approach satisfies the core wound. The inner child is still unseen, praised only through performance, not loved for simply being. True healing comes not from perfecting the false self, but from reconnecting with the Self, the compassionate, curious, and calm internal leader who can turn toward the wounded child, not away from it. Only then can the grandiose protector begin to relinquish its exhausting role, trusting that worth is inherent, not earned through domination, comparison, or applause.

Because the grandiose protective part lacks the flexibility to modulate its behavior according to the nuances and demands of different social environments, it relies heavily on a close collaboration with the chameleon part, a socially attuned protector that displays charm, charisma, and confidence. The chameleon part is skilled at reading the room, masking vulnerability, and adapting to others' expectations to keep the system safe and admired. It helps smooth over the rigid edges of the grandiose part's entitlement, offering an approachable front that earns trust, praise, and belonging.

However, this collaboration is fragile. Beneath the socially polished exterior of the chameleon lies the inflated self-image constructed by the grandiose part. When the chameleon part becomes exhausted or overwhelmed, unable to keep up with the constant emotional labor of managing impressions, the mask begins to slip. In those moments, the underlying grandiose protector steps forward, no longer hidden. Its presence is markedly different: arrogant, cold, controlling, and intolerant of anything that threatens its illusion of superiority.

This shift is often jarring to others. The grandiose part not only demands recognition, approval, and constant compliments, it also expects a passive audience that offers uncritical admiration. It does not engage in mutual dialogue; it seeks to be admired, not understood. While inflated praise and overestimation of performance are welcomed, any constructive feedback is instantly dismissed or attacked. Such feedback pierces the fragile façade and threatens to expose the exiled inner child's deep insecurities and self-doubt.

When confronted with critique, even when offered gently or with care, the grandiose part perceives it as an existential threat. It triggers the activation of the revengeful firefighter, a reactive protector that retaliates through rage, humiliation, or emotional punishment to restore control and suppress vulnerability. The goal isn't simply to reject the feedback, it is to eliminate the discomfort it causes by silencing the source, thereby reinforcing the inner system's illusion of invulnerability.

This protective part seeks to associate itself with individuals perceived as high-status, not only to serve the deeper agenda of the manipulative part, which thrives on social leverage and admiration, but also because being in proximity to such people reinforces a core belief: that only the elite, the powerful, or the exceptionally talented are worthy of their attention or capable of understanding them. In the grandiose protector's worldview, social class is not just about wealth or prestige, it is a reflection of inherent worth. Belonging to this elite group provides the inner child with a sense of specialness, safety, and shared identity, helping to soothe the wounds of early rejection, invisibility, or emotional deprivation.

However, even within these high-status social circles, this part cannot find true rest. After an initial period of admiration or adjustment, where they may feel seen or validated, the grandiose protective part reactivates its drive for dominance and uniqueness. It begins to assess and compare itself to others within the group, unconsciously scanning for threats to its elevated self-image. Soon, admiration turns into rivalry. Rather than finding camaraderie or mutual respect, the grandiose part reinterprets the environment as yet another competitive arena where their worth must be constantly reasserted and proven.

This internal pressure leads to subtle, or sometimes overt, behaviors that disrupt group cohesion: strategic self-promotion, social one-upmanship, attention-seeking gestures, or covert belittling of others who threaten their perceived status. Even among people who outwardly appear aligned with their values or self-image, this part may feel restless or envious when recognition is given elsewhere. In reality, the competition is not only with others but with their own fragile self-concept, which relies on constant external reinforcement to remain intact.

When the grandiose protective part develops in a male inner child, it can manifest through distorted and toxic expressions of masculinity. This part often embodies multigenerational, rigid beliefs about what it means to "*be a man*" - beliefs rooted in domination, emotional repression, and entitlement. These inherited patterns are rarely examined, passed down unconsciously through family systems and reinforced by cultural narratives that equate masculinity with control, superiority, and emotional detachment.

Within this framework, vulnerability is equated with weakness, and power is sought not just socially, but relationally and sexually. The grandiose part may adopt discriminatory attitudes toward individuals who do not conform to heteronormative gender roles, viewing them as inferior or threatening to their fragile internal sense of identity. This part's grandiosity is often propped up by a strict binary: those who affirm their superiority are "real men" or submissive women; those who challenge it are enemies.

In intimate relationships, this part imposes rigid expectations on female partners. Women are perceived not as equals, but as subordinates - caretakers, housekeepers, and emotional support systems. The inner belief is clear: *"She should serve me, admire me, and never challenge me."* Domestic responsibilities and parenting are offloaded onto women, as this part sees these roles as beneath its status. Emotional labor, too, is outsourced - the woman is expected to soothe, sacrifice, and remain silent, even as she is devalued.

In public or social settings, the grandiose part may belittle or dismiss women's perspectives, using humor, mockery, or passive-aggressive comments to assert dominance. It openly expresses entitlement to admiration, physical affection, and preferential treatment, often expecting to be desired without having to give emotional intimacy in return. In professional or financial contexts, it may justify unequal pay or recognition with comments like, "*Men are naturally better at this*," or "*I work harder than most women,*" even when the facts prove otherwise.

At its core, this manifestation of the grandiose part is not about true strength, but a defense against deep-seated fears of inadequacy, invisibility, or rejection. Its toxic masculinity is a mask for a terrified inner child who once believed that being soft, emotional, or dependent would lead to humiliation or abandonment. The grandiose protector steps in to ensure that never happens again, even if it means sacrificing empathy, equality, and connection.

The female grandiose protective part often dominates social interactions, steering conversations toward herself, her accomplishments, and her appearance. Driven by an insatiable hunger for admiration and validation, she becomes highly attuned to flattery, even when it is insincere. Because her focus is so externally driven, she often overlooks or misreads disingenuous praise, mistaking manipulation for admiration. Her sense of self-worth is heavily invested in how others perceive her.

This part frequently adopts roles that cast her as a benevolent leader, organizing charity events, leading community groups, or aligning herself with humanitarian causes, not necessarily out of deep empathy, but because these roles elevate her public image. She wants to be seen as kind-hearted, generous, and admired. Grand gestures are her language of self-importance: hosting elaborate family gatherings, throwing extravagant parties, and giving ostentatious gifts all serve to spotlight her wealth, style, and "perfect" family life. Her carefully curated world, her designer shoes, upscale home, and photogenic family, is not just for her pleasure, but for public consumption and admiration.

Beneath the polished image, however, this protective part maintains a rigid, controlling dynamic with those closest to her. She sees her children not as individuals with unique needs and personalities, but as extensions of her identity. Their accomplishments become her trophies, and their failures, personal insults. She sets unrealistic expectations, urging them to reflect her beauty, intelligence, and ambition. Subtle messages are repeated like mantras: *"You are the best," "You deserve only the finest,"* or *"Never settle for second place."* These affirmations may sound empowering on the surface but mask a deeper belief: that anything short of perfection equals failure. I once witnessed a bedtime ritual in which this part instructed her child to repeat a phrase reinforcing this sense of superiority, almost like a spell.

Because she deems herself either too important or too busy with her career to perform everyday tasks, this part often outsources domestic responsibilities. Nannies, cleaners, or tutors are employed not just for help but as status symbols. Yet those in her service are frequently devalued. She issues orders, criticizes their efforts, and makes disparaging remarks about their backgrounds, whether related to ethnicity, social class, or education. When they fall short of her expectations or assert boundaries, her response is rageful. She cannot tolerate disappointment or defiance without feeling threatened, and she reacts by punishing, belittling, or withdrawing.

Despite the façade of sociability, this grandiose part struggles to form and maintain truly intimate, reciprocal relationships. Her need for admiration overrides the capacity for mutual understanding. Friendships remain superficial; romantic relationships become transactional. She does not share herself; she performs herself. In the end, what appears as confidence is a fragile construct, maintained through constant performance, and protected by entitlement, control, and emotional distance.

I've watched this grandiose protective part orchestrate picture-perfect moments, insisting on posed family photos that showcase a *"cherished memory"* of the flawless family unit. These images are carefully crafted not to preserve authentic connection but to project an idealized narrative: that she is successful, beloved, and surrounded by beauty. The grandiose part thrives on symbols of admiration, so she makes grand gestures in public settings, offering to pay for everyone's meal at the restaurant, leaving generous tips to impress the waitress, or showering friends and family members with expensive gifts. But beneath these acts of generosity lies a strategic intent:

to maintain power through admiration and to reinforce her superior self-image.

Instead of truly valuing fairness, this part covertly demands special treatment, expecting others to yield, accommodate their preferences, or prioritize their needs. Sometimes this is achieved by framing themselves as the most committed, the most oppressed, or the most competent. This part may steal ideas without giving credit, exaggerate its contributions, or present itself as indispensable. It relentlessly seeks validation, needing constant reminders of how valuable, talented, or extraordinary it is.

Ordinary life, to this part, is intolerable. Being *"just another person"* feels like annihilation. To be ordinary is to be unseen, unloved, and shamed. And so, this part keeps striving, chasing recognition, staging perfection, and avoiding vulnerability at all costs. It believes that if it stops performing, it will be discarded. Beneath its shine lies fear, shame, and the buried grief of a child who once felt invisible.

In romantic relationships, the grandiose protective part seeks partners not for emotional intimacy, but for how well they can elevate its public image. Physical beauty, high social status, intelligence, or a prestigious career are all desirable traits - not because they invite emotional closeness, but because they function as extensions of the grandiose part's carefully curated identity. The partner becomes a symbol - a trophy that enhances their social standing, confirming to others (and to themselves) that they are important, superior, and successful.

There is no genuine intention from this protective part to nurture a mutual or emotionally safe connection. Vulnerability is too risky; it threatens the inflated self-image it has built to protect the wounded inner child. Instead, this part controls the narrative, choreographing interactions to maintain dominance and admiration. In public, this part may praise their partner just enough to reinforce the illusion of a perfect union. But in the private realm of their home, where masks can fall away, the grandiose part often reveals its true stance, one of contempt, control, and condescension.

Behind closed doors, the partner is subtly or overtly demeaned, through sarcasm, criticism, emotional invalidation, or outright humiliation. These micro (or macro) aggressions serve a precise function: to diminish the partner just enough to reinforce the superiority of the grandiose part: *"Without me, there is no us."* In these moments, when the partner is belittled or shamed, a euphoric sensation floods the system, a rush of inflated self-worth that briefly soothes the inner child's hidden wounds of inadequacy. A big smile of satisfaction can be seen on their face.

This emotional high, the reward for dominance, acts like a drug. It reinforces the manipulative system's internal logic: *"I am better than you, and therefore I am safe, admired, untouchable."* The partner becomes not a companion, but a mirror whose only function is to reflect the grandiose part's self-image. Any deviation from this role, any assertion of autonomy or criticism, triggers internal chaos: shame, rage, and the retaliatory activation of other protective parts, especially the revengeful firefighter.

Over time, this pattern erodes the relational foundation. The partner may begin to feel invisible, inadequate, or emotionally starved. Meanwhile, the grandiose part doubles down on control, unable to recognize or care about the emotional cost of its behavior. Its mission is not love, but domination dressed as admiration. And as long as the relationship serves that purpose, the grandiose part feels justified, despite the deep, unmet needs it continues to ignore within.

>The high of power courses like a drug,
>I am better, untouchable, admired.
>You are no companion,
>only glass to reflect my crown.
>
>A word out of place, a glance of defiance
>and the fire inside erupts:
>shame, rage, retaliatory sparks
>from hidden guardians I command.
>
>You shrink, fade, become invisible,
>your needs vanish under my throne.
>I double down, blind to the cost,

believing control is love,
while inside, I starve.

4.6 The Inner Critics

You never do enough,
never speak right,
never shine correctly.
Every word I utter,
every step I take,
is weighed and measured
against standards that shift like sand.

The mirror mocks me,
reflecting not what I am,
but what I fail to be.
Even the victories
are tinted with shame,
each success questioned,
each gesture scrutinized.

I hear whispers in the quiet,
voices pointing at flaws,
naming weaknesses I try to hide.
They follow me everywhere,
in the pauses between breaths,
in the half-smile of a friend,
in the fleeting reflection in a window.

And yet, I obey them,
because even in their cruelty,
they feel safe
they keep the chaos at bay,
they remind me to perform,

to please, to survive
in a world that demands perfection.

The inner critics emerge from the inner child's deeply embedded feelings of inadequacy, beliefs forged in the emotional heat of childhood environments where autonomy was sacrificed in exchange for conditional acceptance. These parts were shaped under pressure: manipulated to conform to the expectations of caregivers, punished for authentic expression, and rarely, if ever, affirmed for simply being. As a result, the inner child internalized distorted core beliefs such as: *"I'm not good enough," "I don't deserve love," "I don't deserve success,"* or *"I'm broken and can't change."* The inner critics, though fierce, are protective in nature; they operate in stealth, working in the shadows to ensure the inner child avoids future wounding by preventing risk, failure, or visibility.

4.6.1 The Conformist Inner Critic Protector

Taught to bow
before speaking truth,
trading self
for peace
that never soothed.

A whisper within:
Don't stray. Don't shine.
Love was a cage
disguised
as a shrine.

The conformist inner critic of a self-absorbed person raised in an enmeshed family system develops as a survival strategy, shaped by early experiences where individuality was sacrificed for the sake of family harmony, image, and emotional dependency. In such families, the child is expected to think, feel, and behave in alignment with the caregiver's needs or cultural expectations, often absorbing messages like *"Don't stand out," "Don't question authority," "Family is your top priority"*, or *"We must all agree."*

This protective part supports the inner child's desire to have contact with their family, pressures the inner child to suppress authenticity to maintain emotional proximity and avoid abandonment, shame, or guilt. It polices the self-absorbed person's thoughts and behaviours, harshly criticizing any impulse that could threaten the family's fragile equilibrium or trigger disapproval. The conformist inner critic attacks expressions of autonomy, dissent, or vulnerability, labelling them as disloyal, selfish, or dangerous. Despite its quiet presence, it contributes to a rigid internal system where conformity is mistaken for virtue, and rebellion is equated with betrayal.

The conformist inner critic is relentless and subtle, a part that thrives on maintaining control through obedience and vigilance. It monitors both the other protectors of their inner child and other people, scanning for behaviors that might disrupt the perceived "order" of relationships or family dynamics. In self-absorbed individuals, this critic often collaborates with other protective parts, like the comparer, the dependency critic, or the grandiose protector, to sustain a fragile sense of self-worth built on external approval.

Its voice can be deceptively calm or quietly insistent, whispering warnings like: *"You shouldn't rock the boat," "Your feelings aren't important,"* or *"If you act differently, they'll leave."* Over time, this critic teaches the inner child that safety comes from blending in, minimizing needs, and avoiding confrontation. It discourages vulnerability and authentic self-expression, replacing them with compliance, perfectionism, or over-giving.

Though protective in intention, the conformist critic isolates the person from their own desires, creativity, and self-trust. It convinces them that their value is conditional: only if they are useful, agreeable, and unseen. Ironically, it protects the inner child by teaching them to be invisible, while simultaneously feeding the self-absorbed pattern of control, hierarchy, and judgment in relationships.

> I count my steps, I measure my words,
> a prisoner of nods and sighs.
> To belong is my armor,
> to be myself.

4.6.2 The Comparer Protector

>Always watching,
>never still,
>measuring worth
>against another's will.
>
>Not to love,
>but to outshine,
>to prove:
>*This fragile self is mine.*
>
>But in the race
>to rise above,
>it lost the thread
>of human love.

In many self-absorbed individuals, one of the most active and persistent protectors is the comparer. This part serves as both judge and jury, tirelessly evaluating others to determine whether the person it protects is superior or at risk of being diminished. Its role is not simply to elevate, but to preserve a fragile sense of self-worth built on external validation.

For a self-absorbed person, the comparer functions as a defence against deep-seated shame and insecurity. The comparer arises as a survival strategy, built to protect a child who believed love had to be earned through superiority. But over time, this strategy created a prison of its own, one where connection was sacrificed for image, and where no one, not even the Self, could ever truly be enough. Rather than allow vulnerability or self-reflection, it turns attention outward, scanning for people who appear more successful, more admired, more attractive, so it can either dismiss them, compete with them, or exploit their perceived weaknesses. The comparer thrives on contrast: if someone is seen as inferior, it temporarily soothes the wound of their inner child; if someone is seen as superior, the comparer quickly activates envy, followed by devaluation or strategic imitation.

This protector doesn't seek truth; it seeks control and works closely with the grandiose and manipulative protectors. As any perceived failure or loss in status is intolerable, the comparer immediately generates rationalizations and/or excuses to maintain dominance.

Ironically, while this part tries to protect the inner child from feeling "less than," it also isolates them. Relationships become hierarchical rather than mutual, and emotional intimacy becomes impossible, because the comparer sees others only as threats or pawns, not equals.

> I measure the world in inches and shadows,
> counting victories that vanish by dawn.
> Every face is a mirror I cannot trust
> too bright, and I dim it;
> too dim, and I ignore it.

I tell the child inside,
"You are safe when you stand taller,"
yet I keep the child chained
to the ruler in my hand,
never allowing rest,
never bringing peace.

4.6.3 The Dependency Critic Protector

> Need is a wound,
> it hisses inside,
> softness a threat
> it's sworn to deride.
>
> It built a wall
> from unmet cries,
> and guards it still
> with sharpened lies.

The dependency critic is a fierce inner voice that ridicules and condemns any perceived need for connection, vulnerability, or emotional reliance on others. For the self-absorbed person, this part works closely with the "in control" protective part, being trained by this one to associate dependency with danger, weakness, or humiliation.

It often develops in response to early relational wounds, moments when reaching out for care was met with neglect, ridicule, or manipulation. Rather than risk the pain of rejection again, the dependency critic steps in to sever any emotional need before it surfaces. It whispers harsh messages like *"You don't need anyone,"* or *"Needing help is pathetic."* If the individual finds themselves longing for support, love, or emotional depth, this critic can become brutal, mocking them internally or projecting contempt onto those who express similar needs.

In the internal system of a self-absorbed person, the dependency critic helps uphold the fantasy of emotional self-sufficiency. It reinforces an image of superiority by disowning all vulnerability and by seeing those who express emotional needs as weak, clingy, or flawed. This not only prevents the person from forming authentic bonds but also dehumanizes others, turning emotional connection into a threat to their carefully maintained identity.

The critic arose to ensure that such longing would never surface again, protecting the system from shame, disappointment, and the unbearable grief of unmet needs.

I lock the door
before longing can enter,
and hang a sign that says,
"Need is weakness-keep out."

When the heart whispers for warmth,
I drown it in cold laughter.
I learned long ago
that hands reaching out
can come back empty,
and emptiness is worse than hunger.

So I sharpen my words,
call strength what is really distance,
and stand alone,

safe.

4.6.4 The Doubtful Critic Protector

It doesn't shout,
it waits,
a breath behind belief,
a shadow on the edge
of hope.

It says,
Don't try.
Don't trust.
They'll see you.

So you shrink,
not from failure,
but from the ache
of being known
and still
not enough.

The doubtful critic is one of the most deeply buried and well-defended inner voices in the self-absorbed person's internal system. It is a dominant protective part of vulnerable self-absorbed people, operating from the shadows, whispering self-doubt, planting seeds of hesitation, and sabotaging motivation. It doesn't aim to harm; it aims to *prevent further harm* by keeping the inner child small, invisible, and out of danger. Unlike more obvious critics who shame or ridicule, this one operates in secrecy, often hidden even from conscious awareness. It doesn't shout; it whispers. Its messages are subtle but corrosive, quietly eroding confidence from the shadows, desperately trying to protect the inner child from the pain of failure, humiliation, or rejection.

Because their inner child formed beliefs such as: *"It's safer not to try," "Success will only expose me to attack"*, this protective part questions worth, competence, and belonging, and ignores the evidence that shows their value and abilities. Its voice says things like: *"You'll never be good enough," "Why bother trying?" "You're a fraud", "They'll see through you", "You don't know what you're doing", "You're not good enough to deserve this,"* or *"Someone else will always do it better."* Its goal is to prevent the inner child from being vulnerable again by blocking ambition, numbing dreams, and clouding self-trust. It keeps the system safe by keeping it unseen. When triggered, this part may manifest through procrastination, missed opportunities, self-sabotage, or an inability to celebrate achievements.

But these messages are rarely spoken aloud, not even internally in an obvious way. Instead, they surface as chronic anxiety, indecisiveness, defensiveness, or hypersensitivity to criticism. The self-absorbed person may compulsively seek validation or external proof of their worth, while simultaneously fearing exposure as inadequate.

Because this doubtful inner critic is so threatening to the other protective parts who wish to build an image of superiority for their inner child, it's often disowned. When challenged or confronted, the hidden critic can trigger panic or rage, because even a small crack in the external image risks awakening that buried shame.

Any form of criticism is perceived as a threat to the inner child and is immediately countered. This protector works closely with manipulative parts to deflect blame and avoid accountability. Their common responses include: *"I didn't mean it"*, *"It wasn't me"*, *"I didn't say that"*, *"You made me do it"* or *"You're the narcissist, not me."* Other deflection strategies include circular conversations that never resolve and, of course, silence.

>
> I whisper in shadows,
> "What if it falls apart?"
> "What if you fail?"
>
> I linger at the edges,
> hesitant, vigilant,
> turning every choice
> over in my hands.
>
> Better to warn,
> better to doubt,
> than let the fragile world
> crumble unseen.

4.7 The Scarcity - Minded Protector

Take before it's taken back,
fill the void, avoid the lack.
What if there's not more to gain?
What if wanting ends in pain?

More is safer than enough
love feels scarce, the world is rough.
If nothing's owed, then all is claimed
to need too much is not shameful.

The scarcity mindset protective part operates quietly in the background, often overshadowed by the more dominant manipulative part, yet it holds significant sway over their decisions. Born from the inner child's early experiences of lack of food, safety, affection, attention, emotional connection, and basic stability, this part is deeply shaped by fear.

It emerged as a protective response to unmet needs, internalizing the belief that there is never enough-not enough love, not enough time, not enough resources. Even in times of abundance, it remains convinced that loss is imminent. Its influence shows up subtly, yet persistently, pushing for more accumulation, more control, and more safety through material gain or emotional power.

This part is not inherently greedy; it is afraid. It hoards love, attention, money, and power not out of malice, but out of desperation - desperate to protect the wounded inner child from ever feeling that sense of emptiness again. But in doing so, it often becomes blind to how its choices reinforce cycles of manipulation, disconnection, and fear.

No matter how much love, attention, or reassurance their inner child receives, it is never enough. The scarcity mindset protective part lives in constant fear of loss and abandonment, interpreting anything less than total devotion as rejection. Even minor shifts in attention can ignite intense feelings of abandonment, stemming from the unresolved wounds of their inner child.

This distorted belief, that love must be absolute and exclusive, plays directly into the hands of the manipulative protective part. This part thrives on exclusivity, using emotional tactics to isolate the victim from anything or anyone that threatens their control: close friends, family, hobbies, even pets. Anyone or anything that brings the victim joy, support, or autonomy becomes a perceived threat.

Together, these parts form a dangerous alliance. While the scarcity mindset drives the fear of *not having enough*," the manipulative part acts to *ensure* that no one else can offer the victim what they need. Their combined goal is control, not only over the victim's emotional world but also their financial independence. Restricting access to money, demanding transparency over every cent, and undermining the victim's ability to earn or manage finances are all tools used to reinforce dependency and power.

When the strategies of the manipulative protective part fail to eliminate other "consumers" of love and attention from the victim's life, the fragile system within begins to destabilize. Their inner child, already wired to fear abandonment, perceives the presence of others - whether people, pets - or even the victim's passions, as evidence that they are no longer the center of the victim's world. This perception triggers an acute fear of rejection.

Under this emotional strain, the inner child begins to panic, unable to reconcile the presence of shared affection with its desperate need for exclusivity. The stress doesn't remain contained for long. In response, one of two powerful firefighters may become activated:

- The *revengeful firefighter*, who erupts in rage, seeking to punish the victim for triggering these unbearable feelings. Their tactics can range from verbal abuse and emotional manipulation to financial sabotage and more destructive forms of retaliation.

- Or the *cheater firefighter*, who rushes in to soothe the wounded inner child by seeking admiration elsewhere. Their goal is to restore the illusion of being adored and prioritized, often by pursuing extramarital affairs or emotionally charged connections that offer immediate validation.

Both firefighters serve the same purpose: to restore the emotional equilibrium of the inner child, not through healing, but through short-term coping mechanisms that often come at the expense of others. The love they seek is not grounded in genuine connection, but in control, reassurance, and the illusion of being the only source of someone's affection.

All these emotions and behaviours ultimately create a cycle that closely mirrors the psychological concept of *self-fulfilling prophecies*. The perspectives, desires, and fears of the protective parts, all striving to secure love and attention for their inner child, become deeply intertwined. These parts fuel one another, reinforcing distorted beliefs and responses, and clouding their ability to recognize how their actions cause long-term harm to the very inner child they're meant to protect.

Driven by fear, insecurity, and scarcity, they often act in ways that confirm their worst fears: abandonment, rejection, and inadequacy. Their desperation for love pushes others away. Their fear of betrayal invites secrecy. Their attempts to control create resistance. And their need for validation ultimately leads to emotional disconnection.

Over time, however, the survivors of abuse caused by self-absorbed individuals begin to see through these protective layers. They start recognizing the intentions behind the behaviours. This awareness becomes the seed of transformation. With time and healing, survivors stop reacting to the wounds imposed on them and begin making conscious, empowered decisions. They step out of the cycle, break the prophecy, and choose themselves.

Financial stability offers a wide range of benefits, from better sleep and improved mood to reduced anxiety, increased resilience, and the freedom to plan for the future. Most people strive for it as a foundation for a stable and fulfilling life. The scarcity mindset protective part shares that desire too; it longs to provide the inner child with the safety and comfort they were once denied. However, the way this part pursues financial stability is often shaped not by balance but by fear, and its behaviours can manifest as greed.

No matter how much money is accumulated, it never feels like enough. In the mind of the scarcity protective part, the inner child's worth and sense of security are entirely dependent on financial assets. Stability becomes synonymous with excess. The goal isn't just to have enough to live well, it's to surpass what is needed, as if hoarding wealth can guarantee safety, self-worth, and control over an unpredictable world.

Checking bank balances and watching investments grow brings temporary relief, calming the inner child just enough to sleep through the night. But this comfort is fleeting. As soon as the fear of "*not enough*" returns, whether triggered by an unexpected expense, someone else's success, or a perceived threat to their resources, the cycle restarts, driven by the same wound that was never healed: the fear of lacking, losing, and being left behind.

Before making a new acquisition, the scarcity mindset protective part often crafts a socially acceptable reason, one that seems rational, necessary, or even generous. But beneath the surface lies a deeper, unspoken motive: a persistent, gnawing fear that something will go wrong and their inner child will be left unprotected, hungry, impoverished, or abandoned once again.

The true intention isn't indulgence or luxury; it's survival. Even when the purchase has little to do with basic needs, the protective part is trying to calm an ancient anxiety - the kind born in a home where scarcity wasn't just financial, but emotional, too. This part has learned to mask its fear with logic, to dress its desperation in the language of prudence. But at its core, every acquisition is a form of reassurance - a whispered promise to the inner child: "*You'll never have to go without again.*"

To acquire more money and property, the scarcity mindset protective part is willing to sacrifice not only its own mental and physical well-being, but also that of their partner and children. Fueled by fear and convinced that financial assets are the only true safety net, this part pushes others to overwork, demands better-paying jobs regardless of personal cost, and often scrutinizes, if not outright controls, the household's finances. Any spending outside of bare necessity is framed as reckless, even if it meets emotional or developmental needs.

This protector feeds their children poor-quality food to save more money, has them wear the same clothes for years, and forces younger siblings to wear worn-out hand-me-downs. I can't forget how happy my father was when I decided to cut my hair one day, not because of how it looked or felt, but because it meant he wouldn't have to buy *"so much shampoo."* That moment stayed with me. It wasn't just about shampoo; it was about love measured in savings, affection replaced by control, and a child made to feel like a financial burden.

Most people enjoy offering gifts as expressions of love, appreciation, or simply to bring joy to someone they care about. But for the scarcity mindset protective part, giving is never just about generosity. It resists sharing anything unless there's something to be gained in return. Every interaction is viewed through a transactional lens. If a gift is given, this part ensures its value is clearly communicated in price, subtly guilt-tripping the recipient and setting up an unspoken expectation of repayment. Love, to this part, is not freely given. It must be earned.

Over time, victims of this part's behaviour begin to recognize the strings attached. The joy of receiving is replaced by discomfort, anxiety, and even dread. The memory of genuine appreciation fades, replaced by reminders of sacrifice and obligation.

And yet, this same part feels no hesitation in asking for gifts or favours, especially if they don't involve financial cost to them. Free vacations, complimentary event tickets, or other perks are readily accepted. These gifts satisfy two needs: for the scarcity mindset, they represent a resource gain without expense; for the grandiose protective part, they serve as public validation, proof that they are valued, loved, and important, especially when others are watching. The performance of gratitude matters more than the substance of it.

When the grandiose protective part dominates, the scarcity mindset part steps into the shadows. It doesn't disappear, it quietly observes, keeps count, and tracks every dollar spent in the grandiose part's efforts to impress others. This part may disapprove, but it knows better than to confront the grandiose protector head-on. Instead, it grumbles silently, harbouring resentment over the wastefulness but staying hidden, waiting for a more opportune moment to assert itself.

On the other hand, when the scarcity mindset protective part takes control, the environment becomes guarded and closed-off. Social gatherings, parties, or any activity that might involve spending money are seen as unnecessary risks. The door stays closed, not just to protect their bank account, but to shield the inner child from perceived threats, exposure, comparison, or the obligation to give something in return. In this state, even close family members may find themselves unwelcome, not out of hostility, but because generosity feels like danger.

These two parts, though seemingly at odds, share the same driving force: a deep-rooted fear from childhood. For the grandiose part, love and safety are earned through admiration and status. For the scarcity mindset part, survival comes from control, conservation, and preparation for a world that feels threatening and unstable. Both work tirelessly to serve the same inner child, each believing their strategy is the only way to keep that child safe.

<blockquote>
More, it whispers
more to feel whole.
Stacks of gold
to silence the child.

Worth measured
by what can be owned,
not by what's given
or gently shown.

Yet no matter how much
is claimed or stored,
the vault stays empty
always needing more.
</blockquote>

4.8 The Perfectionistic Protector

> Always producing,
> never enough,
> perfection disguises
> what lies beneath rough.
>
> Achievements stacked
> to silence the doubt,
> chasing applause
> to keep shame out.
>
> Held in a grip
> of tight control,
> afraid of cracks
> that might expose the soul.

Not all the protective parts of a self-absorbed person are loud, destructive, or overtly grandiose. Some self-absorbed individuals present as capable, responsible, and high-achieving on the surface. Behind this polished facade operates a highly functioning and perfectionistic protective part, who is task-oriented, disciplined, and tirelessly driven to maintain order and avoid emotional chaos. This part takes pride in fulfilling societal roles: studying, working, paying bills, managing household tasks. It performs "adulting" with precision, often appearing independent and competent to outsiders. But beneath the surface, it is not the Self who leads, it is a part operating from fear, survival, and desire to bring recognition to their inner child.

The roots of this protector often trace back to rigid family systems where worth was measured by performance. In homes where love was transactional, given only after high achievement, obedience, or perfection, this part was born as a survival mechanism. The message was clear: *"You must earn your place here."* It was also common in families where siblings were pitted against each other for love and attention, and where attention was conditional upon aligning with the caregivers' narrow definitions of success. From such soil, toxic beliefs grew: *"If I'm not busy all the time, I'm worthless," "Only perfection is acceptable,"* and *"My value depends on sacrifice."*

When this part is activated, it operates like a machine. Hyper-focused on outcomes, it drives the system to work excessive hours, overanalyze every detail, and obsessively polish every project. It does this not for personal satisfaction, but in desperate pursuit of the external validation its inner child never received. In this pursuit, it often neglects the emotional, physical, and relational needs. It sacrifices health, friendships, family, and rest on the altar of achievement. And yet, the finish line always moves, the recognition is never enough, the praise never fully lands.

Delegation is especially threatening for this part. Asking for help equates with failure or exposure, as if others might discover how fragile and unworthy the inner child truly feels beneath the image of competence. This resistance to teamwork blocks connection, trust, and collaboration. Even when overwhelmed, they double down, convinced that only they can meet the standard, and that falling short will confirm their deepest fear: that they are fundamentally flawed.

Sometimes, if this part slows down long enough for reflection, the anxiety and exhaustion begin to reveal the unsustainability of its strategy. In rare moments of vulnerability, it may recognize that its constant pushing is not about ambition, but about escaping shame. That awareness, however, is often fleeting, unless held by a compassionate Self or therapeutic relationship that can help it unburden its impossible task.

When the perfectionistic part leads without the support of the Self, life becomes transactional. Tasks replace connection. Schedules become more important than spontaneity. Relationships are measured by usefulness rather than intimacy. This part may tolerate closeness as long as it doesn't interfere with their responsibilities or provoke emotional vulnerability. The inner child, in this system, is exiled, not punished, but ignored, buried beneath to-do lists and achievements.

The emotional needs of their family members, including their inner child, are silenced or pushed aside by this protective part in favor of productivity. Although this protector doesn't seek the spotlight in the same way as the grandiose part, it still wants recognition, just in a quieter, more socially acceptable form. Praise for being competent, self-sufficient, or "*the one everyone can count on*" becomes the emotional currency that feeds this part's engine. Failure, criticism, or any threat to its sense of mastery feels deeply destabilizing, as if the entire system might collapse.

This protector often overidentifies with competence and control in the workplace, building its sense of identity on what it *does*, rather than who it *is*. As a result, it may judge those who seem less organized or driven, projecting internal shame onto others perceived as lazy or emotionally messy. At its core, this part holds fear, fear of failure, fear of judgment, fear of being unlovable without constant proof of worth.

When working in tandem with other self-absorbed protectors, such as the grandiose or perfectionist parts, the highly functioning protector can become hyper-efficient but emotionally numb. It may help construct the illusion of a successful life while suppressing any signals of burnout, loneliness, or inner pain. It resents rest, sees asking for help as weakness, and often neglects basic emotional self-care.

Over time, this part may begin to show signs of fatigue, chronic stress, irritability, anxiety, or even collapse. But instead of slowing down, it pushes harder. Productivity becomes the anesthesia for emotional emptiness.

> Every task must gleam,
> every word must land
> a life composed
> by a trembling hand.
>
> Mistakes are danger,
> mess is defeat,
> so the part runs harder
> to never feel weak.
>
> But inside the grind
> is a plea unheard:
> Am I still worthy
> if I drop the performance?

4.9 The Revengeful Firefighter

I rise like smoke and flame,
a sudden inferno
when the walls are cracked
and shame leaks in.

I strike before they see me,
before the shame touches the small one inside.
Rage is my shield,
vengeance my armor,
and in my heat, the world recoils.

No one notices the child I guard,
the trembling heart behind the blaze.
They only see the fire,
and I let it burn
to keep the secrets safe,
to silence the ache.

The revengeful firefighter gets activated when the protective parts of a self-absorbed person sense that their usual tactics are failing, when their inner child risks losing the victim's love and attention, or faces uncomfortable emotions like shame, rejection, or guilt. In these moments, this firefighter part steps in to sooth the wounded inner child by seeking 'justice' on their behalf. But its idea of justice often mirrors the very abuse the inner child once endured or witnessed. Sometimes, it goes further, finding more subtle or destructive ways to cause harm to the person who triggered those buried wounds.

In a healthy and loving relationship, your partner is your first cheerleader - the one who genuinely wants you to grow, thrive, and achieve your dreams. They celebrate your successes as the result of your hard work and dedication, without seeing themselves in competition with you. But when someone operates from a grandiose protective part, that dynamic shifts. This part struggles to feel genuine pride for another's success and instead becomes agitated by it. The revengeful firefighter, fueled by this part's envy and unresolved anger, reacts from a place of insecurity. Every project, hobby, dream, or even the victim's authenticity becomes a threat, a mirror reflecting the unhealed wounds of their inner child, who once felt unseen, unworthy, and insignificant.

This firefighter is more than just mean; it thrives on creating chaos and inflicting emotional pain. For the revengeful firefighter, hurting others becomes a way to protect the wounded inner child by regaining a false sense of power and control. It will use anything, or anyone, to accomplish this. Its tactics range from subtle to severe. At its lightest, it uses sarcasm, belittling remarks, comments that dismiss or minimize the victim's achievements, or exaggerated focus on their mistakes. But beneath every word is the same goal: to wound others as deeply as the inner child once felt wounded. In severe cases, especially when the abuser lacks empathy, is highly impulsive, and has total disregard for others, the rage triggered by their perceived injury can lead to serious violence, and in rare but real situations, even homicide.

While the chameleon part studies human behavior to mimic empathy and gain acceptance, the revengeful firefighter does the same, but with darker intentions. It observes others carefully, not to connect, but to gather more creative, vengeful tactics and strategies for avoiding accountability. For some, simply recalling the traumatic memories of their inner child is enough to shatter their emotional defenses and awaken this firefighter, whose mission is to make others feel the pain they once endured.

I've witnessed this part emerge - its presence unmistakable in the shift of their eyes - as it fantasized about harming those who had once wounded their inner child or who were now perceived as threats. In those moments, there was no shame, no self-awareness, no regard for how I might perceive them - only the raw, primal drive of a wounded animal craving blood. I've also come to recognize the covert actions of this firefighter part: the one who, in a desperate attempt to soothe the inner child's pain, bad-mouths their victim, leaves damaging reviews under false identities, finds reasons to sue their victim, not only to ruin their reputation but also to serve the scarcity-minded protector who wants to gain financial resources, or even tries to lure their victim back, just to exact revenge on the one who dared to walk away.

To fuel this inner urge, the revengeful firefighter often finds fascination in crime dramas, gangster films, stories of prison life and drug cartels - not for entertainment, but because they mirror its own rage, strategy, and hunger for retribution. These narratives don't disturb them; they validate their worldview.

As tension escalates, the revengeful firefighter may resort to triangulation, weaponizing third parties to amplify the pain of their victim. This third party could be anyone: a child, parent, friend, coworker, someone who has been charmed by the chameleon part's false image. But this tactic goes far beyond mere bad-mouthing. It is part of a calculated effort to destabilize every meaningful aspect of the victim's life.

The revengeful firefighter isn't just vengeful; it is methodical. It can steal money to punish its target, manipulate situations to threaten their livelihood, and actively work to sabotage their career, business, and reputation. It strikes at the victim's sense of safety, aiming to destroy the trust they've built in relationships and communities. No boundary is sacred. Nothing is off limits.

Financial abuse is one of the most insidious tools used by the revengeful firefighter. If the victim has, at any point, shared banking information before an argument or the end of the relationship, this firefighter won't hesitate to exploit it, draining accounts, withdrawing funds without consent, and leaving their victim in a state of shock, panic, and despair.

The revengeful firefighter, driven by rage and a need to restore the illusion of control, may use sex as a weapon. For this part, sexual abuse is not about intimacy - it is about domination, humiliation, and retaliation. It disregards consent, interpreting resistance or silence not as a boundary to respect but as a challenge to overcome. This part may coerce their partner into unwanted sexual acts, using manipulation, threats, or emotional blackmail. Sometimes, the coercion is disguised as a "need for closeness" after conflict. Other times, it appears as forced submission during moments of the victim's emotional or physical vulnerability. In more calculated instances, this part uses sex to reassert dominance after feeling rejected, insecure, or abandoned. The victim may find themselves frozen, dissociating, going along with it in silence, not out of desire, but out of confusion or fear. This silence is later weaponized against them: *"You never said no,"* or *"You stayed, so you must have wanted it."*

To the revengeful firefighter, sexual abuse might be the ultimate tool to reclaim power. It's not always loud or violent. Sometimes, it hides behind closed doors, behind manipulative pleas or twisted justifications. But its impact on the victim is devastating, leaving deep scars of shame, confusion, and betrayal.

This firefighter refuses to pay child support or alimony, weaponizes legal proceedings by intentionally delaying them to drain their victim's resources, and steals valuable items during the separation process. Money becomes a tool for punishment, access is withheld, promises are broken, and assets are hidden to avoid sharing them fairly. Everything becomes transactional, but only on their terms. The goal is not just to win, it's to break their victim down, piece by piece.

The victim's decision to break the cycle of abuse is seen by the grandiose protective part as the ultimate betrayal. It shatters the illusion of control and reactivates the deep abandonment wound of their inner child. The pain that follows feels unbearable, raw, primal, and threatening to their entire internal system.

> Go quietly,
> like dusk dissolving into night.
> Do not pause,
> do not look back,
> or I might reach out.

To retaliate, this firefighter weaponizes their own children, turning them against the other parent without remorse. Their actions strip the children of the love, stability, and consistency every child deserves. In collaboration with the manipulative part, skilled in falsifying information, and the chameleon part, expert at maintaining a false image of a devoted parent, the revengeful firefighter weaponizes the legal system itself. Through prolonged custody battles, they aim to exhaust their victim emotionally, financially, and mentally, all under the guise of protecting the children.

Self-absorbed people rarely forget, and they rarely surrender the illusion of power they believe they hold over their victims. When they sense that control slipping, when silence replaces reaction, they begin to wonder. Has their victim moved on? Has their power truly vanished? This wonder becomes unsettling. It gnaws at their thoughts, distracting them from other parts of their life. Eventually, they reach out again - not out of love, but to test if their victim still responds, still eager to validate their false sense of control. Ironically, in doing so, the self-absorbed person walks into their own trap, revealing how fragile their illusion of power truly was.

This firefighter shows little regard for the consequences of its actions, neither for others nor for its own inner child, whether in the short or long term. Its mantra is stark and unwavering: *win at all costs*. But this mantra is rarely born in isolation; it is often passed down like an heirloom of survival, carried from one generation to the next. I once witnessed a parent reciting it to their child at bedtime, not in those exact words, but in the tone, the warnings, the quiet shaping of belief. Like a nightly prayer, it was whispered into the child's ear: "*Don't let anyone get the better of you. Don't show weakness. Always come out on top.*" In the dark, under the soft hum of a lullaby's rhythm, this seed was planted as misguided love. The child drifted to sleep holding that mantra close, unaware of the heavy inheritance it carried.

However, this firefighter may choose to pause or restrain its destructive impulses when a more calculating protective part recognizes a deeper threat, the risk of losing something profoundly important to the inner child: the carefully curated *public image* crafted and maintained by the grandiose protective part. When that image is at risk of being tarnished, whether through exposure, legal consequences, or social rejection, the firefighter temporarily stands down, not out of remorse, but out of strategy.

> When shame ignites a hidden flame,
> a shadow rises, fueled by blame.
> No wound too small, no slight too thin,
> the fire roars to scorch within.
>
> It lashes out to seize control,
> to wound another, shield the soul.
> A mask of wrath, a blaze of spite,
> a storm unleashed in endless night.

4.10 The Cheater Firefighter

I chase shadows,
seeking warmth in forbidden corners,
a spark to quiet the ache inside.

Every touch, every secret glance,
is a brief reprieve,
a fire to burn away the guilt
that nags,
that whispers
I am never enough.

And when it fades,
I return, hollow and trembling,
to the life I've left smoldering behind.

The cheater firefighter emerges in the self-absorbed internal system as a reactive, impulsive part whose core purpose is to numb, soothe, or escape overwhelming internal pain. This part is not inherently malicious or immoral, it exists as a last resort, an emergency responder to the deep unmet needs and insecurities of the inner child. When unbearable feelings of inadequacy, rejection, emotional starvation, or vulnerability are triggered, this part rushes in with the only tool it knows: distraction through the excitement of sexual or romantic conquest.

In many self-absorbed individuals, the cheater firefighter is activated by internal dissonance. For example, when the grandiose part fails to meet its expectations of admiration, or when the perfectionist part is criticized despite all its efforts, the exiled inner child is left exposed, flooded with shame, worthlessness, or loneliness. In those moments, this firefighter floods the system with impulsive urges, chasing short-term gratification to override long-term emptiness. The act of cheating, whether emotional, physical, or even digital, is not about love or attraction. It is about sedation.

The cheater firefighter often operates in secrecy, bypassing the moral constraints imposed by more managerial parts. It creates an illusion of empowerment, control, or desirability, allowing the self-absorbed individuals to reclaim a sense of superiority that has been threatened. It whispers seductive narratives: *"You deserve better," "They don't appreciate you,"* or *"You're still desirable."* These stories serve as protective buffers against the raw pain of feeling insignificant, unloved, or unseen.

This part is often fueled by a distorted narrative about intimacy and worth. In self-absorbed systems, intimacy is not experienced as safe or nourishing, it is experienced as conditional, suffocating, or even dangerous. Early enmeshment, emotional manipulation, or betrayal by caregivers may have shaped the belief that closeness leads to control or vulnerability. Therefore, cheating becomes a paradoxical way of asserting independence. It gives the illusion of agency while avoiding the risk of deep emotional exposure.

In some systems, this firefighter collaborates with the grandiose part, reinforcing the belief that the self-absorbed individual is too exceptional to be confined by loyalty. In others, it acts out against the perceived entrapment imposed by the perfectionist or conformist parts, which demand emotional performance in relationships. True intimacy activates the buried wounds of the inner child, and this part would rather escape than feel.

Despite its explosive actions, the cheater firefighter is often followed by a wave of guilt, denial, or emotional disconnection. The system quickly rushes to protect itself, minimizing the impact, blaming others, or rationalizing the behavior. The inner critics may awaken afterward, attacking the individual with shame-laced accusations, only to push the firefighter back into action in a painful, self-perpetuating cycle. This looping dynamic reinforces the emotional isolation that lies at the core of their inner child's wounding.

Partners and loved ones often feel deeply confused by the presence of this part. On the surface, the self-absorbed individual may appear invested in the relationship, loyal, charming, or even attentive. Yet behind the mask, the cheater firefighter exists in a different reality, one governed by impulse and emotional avoidance rather than commitment. Attempts by the partner to confront or express pain are often met with gaslighting, deflection, or the cold withdrawal of the emotional manager parts.

In therapy, this firefighter is one of the hardest parts to access and understand, as it is steeped in shame and avoidance. It hides behind the justifications of the manipulative protective part and rarely trusts that anyone could witness its actions without condemnation. However, when met with compassion and curiosity, this part can begin to reveal the truth: it is not the source of the problem, but a symptom of deep emotional wounding. It carries the burden of trying to soothe pain it did not create.

> I run down alleys of desire,
> looking for a door
> to swing open
> and let the pain escape.
>
> I lie to myself,
> telling the small one inside:
> "It is only temporary.
> It keeps the world from collapsing."
>
> But the relief is fleeting,
> and the shadow follows me home,
> long after the fire dies.

4.11 The Self of a Self-Absorbed Person

> I am the quiet pulse beneath the storm,
> the small voice drowned
> by shields, masks, and fire.
>
> I watch the grandiose parade,
> the chameleon slip into every shape,
> the firefighters flare and vanish.
>
> I am here,
> hidden and unnoticed,
> waiting for a glance inward,
> a moment to be known.

Every person has a Self. It is present from the very beginning, quietly witnessing the journey of the inner child, guiding with kindness, compassion, creativity, persistence, honesty, and love. In difficult times, when our protective parts struggle to meet the needs of the inner child, the Self continues to offer guidance. These parts may have free will, but they are never alone; the Self is always offering direction, however softly.

The Self of a self-absorbed person, like in all people, remains intact beneath layers of protective and wounded parts. It is calm, compassionate, connected, and curious, qualities often obscured by the complex inner system developed in response to deep emotional injuries. But in self-absorbed individuals, the Self is rarely permitted to lead. It is not because it is absent or broken. Rather, over time, protective parts have disconnected from their Self, as they started gravitating around dominant protector parts, like the grandiose, manipulative, or perfectionistic ones.

These protective parts formed in the face of overwhelming emotional threats, moments when the inner child felt unseen, unloved, or utterly powerless. Perhaps, in these moments of vulnerability, the system determined that sensitivity was dangerous, authenticity was unsafe, and the open-heartedness of the Self could not be trusted to keep the system alive. So, protectors rose up: the grandiose part inflated the child's worth to compensate for their invisibility; the manipulative part learned to read and control others to ensure survival; the perfectionist drove relentless achievement to stave off the unbearable pain of not being good enough. Each took on a sacred duty, believing they alone could protect the most fragile parts of the system.

When we disconnect from the Self, our protective parts lose access to that quiet, steady voice. They grow accustomed to ignoring it, especially when it reminds them not to cross boundaries or cause harm. The Self never condones mistreatment. It gently warns, helps us see the consequences of our actions, and invites us back to alignment, again and again. As these protectors solidify their roles, the Self is pushed into the background, because it is misunderstood. The protectors see the Self's calmness as weakness, its openness as a threat, its patience as passivity. To them, control, image, and strategy are safer. Over time, they built a fortress of activity, performance, and distortion, distancing themselves from the one inner presence that could truly bring them home.

And so, the Self becomes a whisper, present, yet unheard. It watches the protectors exhaust themselves in pursuit of validation, in desperate attempts to avoid shame, in cycles of control and collapse. It waits through tantrums, illusions, and retreats. It does not interfere, because the Self does not dominate, it invites. It does not punish, it welcomes.

Even when protective parts pull away, distancing themselves from its presence, the Self remains. Watching. Waiting. Always ready to be seen and heard. It quietly waits beneath the chaos, capable of witnessing without judgment, leading without domination, and healing with truth and love. At times, when these protective parts are relaxed, the Self is present, showing them the beauty of others, without triggering jealousy, of the waterfalls, and the ocean.

For self-absorbed individuals, reconnecting with the Self is not a linear path. It requires a system-wide reckoning, a compassionate confrontation with the truth: that the parts who led the way were only doing so to protect a deeply wounded child. These parts must first be met with empathy, not exile. They must be invited to see that the Self is not their enemy, but the very source of the love, clarity, and healing they have always longed for.

When self-absorbed individuals begin to turn inward with genuine curiosity and openness, their Self can begin to emerge, not to shame the parts, but to guide them home. True transformation begins not by destroying the protective system of the inner child of a self-absorbed person, but by helping the protectors trust that the Self is strong enough to lead.

The journey back to Self is both terrifying and liberating. Terrifying, because it means relinquishing control and facing the wounds that formed long ago. Liberating, because the Self carries no judgment, only presence. When the protectors begin to trust this presence, they soften. They speak more honestly. They begin to rest.

And in this sacred resting, the internal system of a self-absorbed, once built to defend and dominate, can finally begin to heal.

I see the games,
the mirrors, the clever disguises.
I see the thirst for admiration,
the hunger for control,
the fear behind every move.

I am not them,
yet I live inside them,
bearing witness to all
while trying to remember
who I truly am.

Conclusions

Healing, I've come to understand, is not a final destination. It is not something we achieve, complete, or master. Rather, it is a lifelong process of remembering, reuniting, and reclaiming. It is the slow, often messy, and always courageous work of turning inward, again and again, to meet the parts of ourselves that have waited in silence for love, safety, and acknowledgment.

This memoir captures one chapter of that ever-evolving journey. It reflects a time when I dared to stop running from my pain and instead chose to sit with it, to listen, to trace its roots back to childhood, back to the familial patterns and emotional imprints that shaped my sense of self. I initiated my healing through honest conversations with my inner world. It was in the quiet presence of my Self that I began to see the truth: that I had never been broken - only burdened, fragmented, and shaped by the wounds of my ancestors.

In writing this story, I reclaimed more than just my voice. I honoured the many parts of me that had long struggled in isolation - the overgiver, the inner critics, the highly functioning, the one "in control", the risk manager, the warrior, the doubter, the child who simply wanted to be seen. Each of these parts emerged not to harm but to protect my inner child in the only ways they knew how. They were forged in the fires of survival, shaped by abandonment, neglect, and confusion. And yet, they carried wisdom. When I stopped rejecting them and began relating to them with compassion and curiosity, something remarkable shifted: they softened. They trusted and evolved.

This is what it means to heal from the inside out. Not to erase the past or deny the pain, but to integrate it - to transform it by walking through it with presence and patience. My protective parts no longer carry their burdens alone. They are no longer trapped in outdated roles. They now work with my Self, not against it. Together, we've created an inner ecosystem built on trust, attunement, and respect.

Professionally, I understood how trauma fragments the inner system. But it was only through lived experience that I came to know how true healing happens - how love, not logic, is what brings our parts home. It is not analysis that restores us, but relationships. Self-energy - that calm, connected, wise essence within - is what rebuilds what trauma once splintered.

Spiritually, this healing has felt like a homecoming. I came to recognize that the Universe had always been speaking to me through synchronicities, dreams, and inner nudges. I simply wasn't yet ready to listen. The signs I once ignored became symbols of support. The detours I once resented became teachers. I no longer see the people who hurt me as proof that I was unlovable, but as mirrors showing me where I had abandoned myself.

There is a stillness at the center of every human being, a place untouched by fear, chaos, or rejection. Whether we call it Self, soul, divine essence, or intuition, that presence remains. It waits, quietly, patiently, until we are ready to return. And when we do, it welcomes us without judgment.

This process is ongoing. There is no endpoint. Writing this memoir is not the final chapter, but a meaningful milestone in a lifelong journey. I still experience grief. I still pause before making decisions, aware now that hesitation is not a flaw, but a sign of self-respect - of checking in with all the parts within me before acting. I have no desire to be perfect and I no longer strive to rescue others. My healing is an everyday practice.

The child within me, the one who longed to be heard, held, and loved , finally has a seat at the table and my protectors no longer expect epiphanies to fix everything. They no longer run the show in fear. They move with greater patience and wisdom, each step forward a gesture of love rather than urgency.

Today, I can say with unwavering truth: I have come home to myself. The voice of my heart is clear now: I am whole in my imperfection. I do not have to abandon myself to be loved. I do not have to explain my worth. I do not have to carry others' healing on my back. I no longer believe I hold the key that brings light to others' darkness. Each person carries their own key and each must choose to turn it. I hold compassion for those I've loved, including those who were emotionally unavailable, self-absorbed, or lost in their own pain. But I no longer believe that compassion means shrinking myself or sacrificing my truth. The people in my life who embodied self-absorption traits were not the destination, they were messengers. They pointed me toward the places within that still needed attention, integration, and grace. They catalyzed my return, but they are no longer the center of my story.

As I look back over my journey, I see not just my own healing, but the unraveling of threads woven generations before me, threads of silence, shame, and unhealed wounds passed down like an unspoken inheritance. I have chosen to be the one who breaks this chain out of love for myself and for those yet to come. Healing, I have learned, is not just a personal act; it is an offering to the future, a quiet promise that the story can be told differently. My hope is that the generations that follow will walk further along this path, not burdened by the same wounds, but guided by the wisdom, compassion, and self-love that have taken root here. If my life can be a bridge between what was and what can be, then every step into my own wholeness has been worth it.

I am home.

Bibliography

1. Angelou, Maya. *I Know Why the Caged Bird Sings*. Random House, 1969.
2. *A Course in Miracles*, Combined Volume (Third Edition), (Mill Valley, CA: Foundation for Inner Peace, 2007), Text, Ch. 16, Section IV, para. 6.
3. Carl G. Jung, *Aion: Researches into the Phenomenology of the Self* (Princeton: Princeton University Press, 1968), para. 126.
4. Maya Angelou, quoted in Marcia Ann Gillespie, Rosa Johnson Butler, and Richard A. Long, *Maya Angelou: A Glorious Celebration* (New York: Doubleday, 2008), 167.

www.ingramcontent.com/pod-product-compliance
Lightning Source LLC
Chambersburg PA
CBHW050344010526
44119CB00049B/695